Baby Sleep Solution

2021 Edition

Gentle Ways to Help Your Baby Sleep Through the Night, the No Cry Sleep Solution for Newborn and Toddler, the Advanced Guide for Parents

Gerarld Paul Clifford

described as a work of fiction. Regardless of the nature of this work, the Publisher is exempt from any responsibility of actions taken by the reader in conjunction with this work. The Publisher acknowledges that the reader acts of their own accord and releases the author and Publisher of any responsibility for the observance of tips, advice, counsel, strategies and techniques that may be offered in this volume.

Table of Contents

Chapter 6: Teaching Them to Wind Down 75

Chapter 7: Have a Great Nap 88

Chapter 8: Sleep Schedule........................... 101

Chapter 9: Sleep Issues 116

Conclusion 132

Introduction

Thank you for choosing this book. I hope that you find the information within this book helpful and informative. This book will discuss different ways to help your child get a good night's sleep. Sleep is essential for everybody, so it's important to teach your child early on how to get and stay asleep.

We'll start by going over how to set up a baby's room to help them have a good night's sleep, as well as a safe sleep. Having the right setting can make or break your newborn's sleep quality, so if you have it right at the start, you'll have less to worry about later on.

Then we will move into looking at sleep tricks for newborns up to three months old. This is when parental sleep deprivation can kick in, but we'll go over how to help your baby sleep better at night so that you don't have to worry about it.

Then we'll move into the three to six-month period. Here is when your baby is going to start sleeping more, which will give you time to catch up on your sleep. Next, we'll finish up looking at the first year of life with six to 12 months old. We'll look at changes that may happen to sleep due to teething and how to work through those issues.

After that, we'll discuss what sleep with a toddler will look like. This will discuss one year to five years old and how their sleep will change from when they were a baby.

Then we'll move into teaching children how to wind down before bed. We can all use some time before bed to calm down and relax the body and mind to help us drift off to sleep. If you can teach your child how to do this on their own, it can make your life a lot easier.

Next, we'll talk about how to help your child have a great nap, and then we will look at coming up with a sleep schedule. Sleep schedule is one of the most effective tools in the parent's arsenal to ensure your child sleeps well.

Lastly, we will talk about sleep issues. Sometimes your child not wanting to sleep is caused by an actual problem that they need help with. When you know what to look for, you can get ahead of it before it becomes a significant problem.

With that said, let's get into the information you came here for.

Chapter 1: Setting the Scene

The first step in helping your baby sleep is making sure their room is set up correctly. This serves two purposes. One is that having the wrong setup can actually hurt a baby. Two is that the right atmosphere can help a baby's sleep. Our first stop is looking at a proper and safe set up to make sure your baby sleeps safely.

Safe Nursery Setup

Over 3500 babies die suddenly each year in the US, often caused by SIDS or accidental death due to strangulation or suffocation. To try and lower the risk of deaths during sleep, the AAP (American Academy of Pediatrics, came up with guidelines for what you should and should put in your baby's room. The following are tips from the AAP to ensure your baby stays safe at night.

1. Place Them on Their Back

Up until the first birthday, a baby needs to sleep on their back for all sleep times. Research has found that babies who are placed on their backs have a lower chance of dying from SIDS than those who are placed on the sides or belly. The issue that arises when you place them on their sides is that they could roll onto their belly. Some believe that babies may end up choking when they sleep on their backs, but the way their anatomy is made, and their gag reflex, will prevent anything like that from occurring. Even babies who have been diagnosed with GERD can safely sleep flat on their backs.

There will come a time when baby rolls to their belly. If you know they can move from back to belly and back again, then they are fine and there is no need to move them back to their back. However, you need to make sure you don't have any pillows, blankets, bumper pads, or stuffed toys around them. This will ensure that they won't roll into them, which may smother them.

If they were to fall asleep in their carrier, sling, swing, stroller, or car seat, you should place them onto a firm surface on their back as soon as you can.

2. Keep a Firm Sleep Surface

It is strongly recommended that you use a play yard, portable crib, bassinet, or crib that meets the CPSC safety standards. In it, you should place a firm, tight-fitting mattress with fitted sheets that is supposed to go in there. Nothing else should be place in the crib other than the baby. Having a firm surface does not mean it has to be a hard surface. However, the bed should not indent when you lay the baby down. You may see commercials for mattresses or sleep surfaces that are said to lower the risk of SIDS, but there isn't any evidence that has proven those statements. If they meet the CPSC standards, you can still use them.

3. Only Allow Baby in Your Bed to Comfort or
Feed

When your baby is ready to sleep, make sure, you place them in their own sleep space. While you do have your baby in your bed while feeding or comforting them, make sure that you don't have any blankets, sheets, pillows, or other items that could cover their neck, face, and head if you were to fall asleep. If you do fall asleep, once you wake up, move your baby into their own sleep space.

4. Bed Sharing Should Not Be Done for Any Baby

You should never share your bed with your baby because it is dangerous. There are things that can make sharing a bed even more hazardous. Never share the same bed with your baby if:

- If any person in the bed is a smoker
- They are under four months old
- The mother smoked while pregnant
- You consumed alcohol
- You aren't the baby's parent
- You are on a soft surface like an armchair, couch, sofa, old mattress, or waterbed
- You took something before bed that can affect your ability to wake up
- There is soft bedding on the bed
- They had a low birth weight or was premature

5. Share The Room with Your Baby

It is sometimes a good idea to sleep in the same room with your baby for at least the first six months, if not for the first year. You can place the crib or bassinet near your bed. The AAP has said that it is a good idea to share the room with your baby since it can reduce the risk of SIDS by 50%, and is much safer than having them in bed with you. Plus, room sharing makes watching, comforting, and feeding your baby easier.

6. Loose Bedding and Soft Objects Should Be Kept Away from Them

You need to keep things like loose bedding, toys, bumper pads, sheepskins, comforters, quilts, and pillows. These things can increase the risk of suffocation, entrapment, or strangulation. If you are worried that they may get cold, use infant clothing to help keep them warm, like a wearable blanket. Typically, you should dress your baby in only one layer more than what you have on.

7. Don't Let Them Sleep on Lounge Pads or Nursing Pillows

Babies could end up rolling onto their stomachs or sides and then their head gets pressed into the soft surface. Or, if they are propped on a lounger or pillow, the head can fall forward, which will block their airway. Between 2012 to 2018, more than two dozen infants died after they were left near or on those types of products.

8. Give Pacifier at Nap and Bedtime

Giving them a pacifier when sleeping can help to lower SIDS risk, even if they drop it once they fall asleep. If you breastfeed, wait until you are done before you offer them a pacifier.

Creating a Sleep Sanctuary

Let's face it; sleep is probably one of the best things when it comes to having a baby. With early-morning soothing and late-night feedings and everything in between, it's important to create a sleep conducive space. You need a room that is dark when it should be, light whenever you need it, warm and comfortable for both you and your child.

While you may also be interested in color schemes, rugs, and crib styles, your babies are not going to care too much about those things. We're going to look at some ways to bring all your hard designing work together to make a place that will help your baby sleep and possibly give you a few more hours of z's as well.

Temperature

Do you worry that the sleep environment could be too cold or too hot for your baby? That makes sense and is an essential thing to consider. They have also found links to overheating and SIDS, so it is better to be safe than sorry. The best temperature to shoot for is between 68 and 72 degrees. Babies can't adapt to temperature changes in the same way adults can. You should go with your gut to figure out if your baby is too hot or too cold, but the following information can help you decide.

1.   Signs It's Too Cold

If you touch your baby's nose or hands and they are
cool to the touch, that may not be anything to worry
about. However, if you feel the chest area and it is
cold, then they are probably too cold. If you notice
that their lips have turned blue, they are definitely too
cold. If you are worried that their room may be too
cool, go ahead and put an extra layer on them, like an
onesie under pajamas.

2.   Signs It's Too Hot

If your baby has a fast heart rate, damp hair, or is
sweating, they are too hot and need to be cooled off.
You should always be safe and don't let worry override
your common sense. Keep space heaters out of your
baby's room and especially away from window
coverings.

Lighting

Just like adults do well sleeping in the dark, babies do
too. Our sleep hormones are released in the dark, so
even science tells us that it is best to sleep in a dark
room. When you make the baby's room dark, think of
it as a cave. The goal here is to be able to make your
baby's room dark at any point in the day, even when it
comes to napping, because parents can get some sleep
then too.

While you may be worried that getting your baby used
to sleep in such a dark room will make it hard for
them to sleep anywhere else, don't worry. I can ensure

that your child will still be able to sleep in less than perfect sleeping conditions like daycare or the car.

Blackout coverings or shades are a great way to turn your baby's room into a cave. Don't worry about it costing you a fortune to get those coverings. In fact, let's go over some cheap ways to make the baby's room dark.

First, you don't have to go for curtains right off the bat. You can take some construction paper or cardboard and tape it to the windows with some blue painter's tape to keep the light out. Make sure that you check for condensation so that you don't start growing mold.

You can also get cellular blackout shades, which can be custom fit for your windows. These do cost more than some blackout shades or the DIY version we just covered, and they also aren't super expensive. Cellular shades also have thermal properties that can help to reduce your cooling and heating costs, so they can help pay for themselves. However, there is a sliver of light that will come out from the sides of the shades because you can't get a flush fit, so you aren't going to get cave dark.

Lastly, you have BlackoutEZ covers. They are affordable, custom fit, and they look great. Plus, they are going to seal out all of the light so that there is nothing that gets through. These would probably be the best option, in my opinion.

Sound

It's easy to wake up a baby with a sudden sound. To make a sleep environment for your baby that will teach them good sleep habits, think about getting a white noise machine for their room. The white noise machine will remind them of the noises they heard in their womb. This noise will comfort them, and it was actually quite loud. Go ahead and plug the machine in to recreate that special environment.

There are a lot of white noise machines out there on the market, but are they all worth the price? Dohm is considered to be the best. It has a fan that creates its signature sound, unlike others that use electronic sounds. They also have a mini-travel version. If you want a cheaper option, you can't really go wrong with any other white noise machine you find. Homedics has a white noise machine that is really good and affordable.

When it comes to a white noise machine, you should focus on only using white-noises. There are plenty of sound machines out there that can play things like an ocean breeze and rainstorms, but white noise is the best for you, baby. Other types of noise can end up stimulating their brain activity while sleeping.

Those are the three main things you need to think about, but let's go over some things you may want to consider.

1.   Personal preference

For decades, nurseries have been dominated by two things: cute and things that clean up easily. Now people have started to move away from pastel colors and a utilitarian focus to picking something that the parents actually enjoy. This could be a theme that reminds you to have your own childhood or artwork that would be appealing to the baby and you.

2.   Comfort

You want to be happy with the way it looks, but you should also like the way it feels. You are going to be spending a lot of time there. Having a comfortable rocking chair is great whether you breastfeed or not. Anybody who takes care of the baby will get good use out of a comfy rocking chair. You can add pillows and blankets to the chair to make it more comfortable for you. You being comfortable is going to help your baby as well.

3.   Function over form

This room gets a lot of use. It isn't just a place where your baby sleeps, so it's important to keep it organize the best you can. You are going to have to be able to find things at night while still half-asleep. It's better to have things that function well in the room that you can get to with ease than those that look "cute" but doesn't help you do anything.

4.   Colors

Color preference may be up to the parents at this point, but you should avoid any type of contrasting or intense colors and patterns. Once the baby can see colors, contrast can stimulate their brain. While it's fine to have educational things on the walls, such as shapes, pictures, numbers, and letters, it helps create a least one neutral area of the room where they can shift their focus.

Creating a safe and sound environment for your baby to sleep in is an important step in making sure that you both get the sleep you deserve. You don't have to spend a bunch of money to do this either. There are affordable white noise machines and blackout shades that can help your baby create a calming environment. And make sure you don't buy into the hype of a product that is meant to help your baby sleep better. Chances are, it won't be safe to have in the crib with them; it will probably cost a fortune, and it likely won't work. You know your baby better than anybody else does, so go with your gut.

Chapter 2: Birth to Three Months: Helping Them Sleep

Newborn babies will sleep anywhere from 11 to 18 hours every day, and this gets done during all hours of the day and night. They won't sleep for more than a couple of hours at a time because they need to be fed frequently. This means you are going to have some sleepless nights in the beginning. Their sleep patterns might be very unpredictable for a bit, but there isn't any need to put them on a sleep schedule just yet. There are some things that you can do to help them develop good sleep habits.

This is a normal phase that your baby has to go through, but the good news is, it won't last too long. Even though to an unrested mom, it might seem like an eternity.

A baby's sleep cycle is a lot shorter than an adult's. They are going to spend more time in REM sleep, which can be easily disturbed. This is needed for the changes in their brains.

By the time they are six to eight weeks old, they might sleep for shorter periods during the day and for longer at night. They are still going to wake up to be fed during the night, but they will have more deep periods of sleep with fewer light nights of sleep.

It might be possible that your baby will sleep through the night at eight weeks old, but this is not typical. Each baby is different, and your nights will probably get interrupted for the first few months. If you want to get your baby to sleep through the night, you need to encourage some habits from the beginning.

Typical Sleep Schedules

Even though newborns will sleep anywhere from 11 to 18 hours every day, they might not sleep, but a few hours each time they go down for a nap.

During these first three months, they will start to sleep longer, but many infants won't sleep more than a four or six-hour time period.

Here is what a two-month-old baby's sleep schedule might look like:

- Wake up – 6:30 AM
- Sleep – 8 to 10:30 AM
- Wake up, feed, play – 10:30 AM to 12 PM
- Sleep – 12 to 3 PM
- Wake up, feed, play – 3 to 9 PM (might have some naps during this time)
- Sleep, wake up to feed – 9 to 11:30 PM
- Sleep, wake up to feed – 12 to 3:30 AM
- Sleep, wake up to feed – 4 to 6:30 AM

This is just an example, and your baby might not sleep like this. Your baby might sleep at different amounts of time according to your activities and schedules.

A sleep schedule for a three-month-old is going to be different from a two-month-old. There isn't a specific sleep schedule that a three-month-old should follow. Many three-month-olds will sleep several times throughout the day to reach 18 hours. There will be some differences between a sleeping pattern of a newborn and a three-month-old.

By the time a baby reaches three months old, they will sleep for longer periods of time during the night and shorter times during the day. Basically, a three-month-old will sleep about seven and a half hours at night.

Three-month-olds are more likely to wake up less during the night than a newborn. Basically, a three-month-old will only wake up about three times each night; this is a lot less than a newborn.

Unpredictable Sleep Patterns

Why do newborns have unpredictable sleep patterns? Babies typically don't have a good sleep pattern until they are about three months. Their circadian rhythm has not be developed, which controls when they should be awake and when they should sleep. It runs 24 hours a day and turns off and on at regular intervals between alertness and sleep.

Nutritional needs might cause unpredictable sleep patterns. You might need to feed your baby every two to three hours during their first month. It might change in their second month to being fed every three to four hours. As they get older, they won't require all of those night time feedings.

The good news is those unpredictable sleep patterns will stop. It might seem like forever for a sleep-deprived mom. Some babies will sleep for longer periods by the time they are three months old. Others won't until they are older.

Pregnancy Sleep Patterns

Will the sleep pattern my baby developed during pregnancy continue once they are born? You might have heard a rumor that if your baby is active at night during pregnancy that they will be a night owl once they are born. Some moms say this is true, but there isn't any scientific evidence that states otherwise. Yes, your baby will develop a sleep-wake cycle before they are born. When your third trimester starts, they will begin having REM sleep. This is when a person dreams during their sleep. They will begin having non-REM about a month later.

Babies in utero won't have our normal day and night schedules, just like newborns won't. They will rest for a couple of hours, and then they will wake up for a couple of hours.

Day and Night Means Nothing to Babies

Babies won't develop the knowledge of knowing when day is and when night is until they are about one month old. How much sleep they get at night will be about the same as what they get during the day. This might be anywhere from six weeks to three months. Their melatonin and body temperature will help them begin developing a different sleep-wake cycle during the day and night.

Baby's Sleep Cycles Differ From Adults

A baby's sleep cycle will be a lot shorter than an adult's sleep cycle. A newborn's sleep cycle will be in REM sleep about have the time. Adults or older children will spend a lot less time in REM sleep. Some have come to believe that newborns have to have a lot of REM sleep since it helps with brain development Newborns have what is equal to REM sleep, known as "active sleep," since their eyes will move underneath their eyelids. Their legs and arms might jerk or twitch during sleep, too. They will transition into a quieter sleep where twitches stop, their breath becomes deeper, and it's harder to wake them up. They might switch between REM and non-REM cycles several times during their sleep.

Do Newborns Need A Sleep Schedule?

During the first few weeks of like, they don't need a schedule since their sleep patterns are irregular. This mostly happens because they need to sleep and eat a lot during this time.

You can begin following some sort of schedule during these first few months by creating nap times and a specific bedtime. As they begin sorting out their sleep rhythms, creating these kinds of routines already in place while introducing good sleep habits could help them settle into a schedule as they get older. Going outside during the day, especially during morning hours, can help them begin getting into a better schedule.

Do I Need To Wake Them To Feed Them?

Not after the first few weeks. Talk to your baby's doctor to see if you need to wake them. It is generally fine to allow them to sleep for longer stretches without feeding them.

It all would depend on how well your baby is feeding and growing, especially if they lost some of their birth weight. Normal babies will lose some weight in the first few days after birth but will gain it back by two weeks old. Their doctor might recommend you wake them every few hours until they are back to their birth weight.

If your baby is gaining weight and growing, eating well, and having plenty of poopy and wet diapers for their age, their doctor might say that it is fine to let them sleep for longer periods of time. Most younger babies will wake up hungry in a few hours.

Can You Teach Newborns Good Sleep Habits?

Sure, but you need to do it slowly and don't expect them to learn fast. Babies can develop good sleep habits from about six weeks old. This is when they will begin developing their circadian rhythms. Here are a few ways to settle your baby.

- Allow Them To Take Frequent Naps
During their first eight weeks, most babies aren't going to be awake for long than a couple of hours, if that. If you make them stay awake longer than that, they might get too tired and have problems getting to sleep.

- Show Them The Difference Between Night and Day
Some babies are going to be wide awake at night when you are ready to go to sleep, while others are early birds. You aren't going to be able to do anything about this for the first few weeks. Once they reach two weeks, start teaching them about the difference between night and day.

  - Daytime
    - Change their clothes when they wake up. This helps them understand that it is the beginning of the day
    - Interact, play, and talk to them as much as you can

- Make their feedings during the day social. Talk to them while you are feeding them
      - Keep their room and house bright
      - Allow them to hear the daytime noise like the dishwasher, washing machine, vacuum, television, or radio.
      - If they nod off during feeding, wake them up gently
  o Night
      - Bathe them
      - Put them into their pajamas to show them that daytime is over and it is time to sleep
      - Don't talk to them while you are feeding
      - Keep the noises off
      - Light needs to be very low

All of these things should help show your baby the differences between night and day.

- Know When Your Baby is Tired

For about the first six weeks, your baby might not be able to stay awake for more than a couple of hours. If you wait too long, they might become too tied and won't go to sleep easily. You are going to develop a strong sense about their sleeping patterns. You'll know once they are ready to sleep. If you spot any signs that they are sleepy, try to put them to bed as quickly as you can.

During their first three months, you need to be able to recognize their sleepy signs like easily:

1. Getting still and quiet
2. Losing interest in toys or you
3. Stretching or yawning
4. Staring into space
5. Crying or whining
6. Dark circles under their eyes
7. Flicking or pulling their ear
8. Rubbing their eyes

They might turn away from you or moving objects. They could bury their face against your chest. If you see any of these signs, put them down as soon as you can. You will soon become familiar with their patterns and cues that show you they are ready for a nap.

- Begin a Bedtime Routine

You can never start a bedtime routine too early. This might include some simple things like:

- Bathing them
- Change their diaper and clothes
- Feed them
- Sing them a song or play some soft music
- Kiss them goodnight

- Put Them To Bed While Awake but Sleepy

By the time your baby is six to eight weeks of age, you can begin trying to give them a chance to fall asleep by themselves by laying them in their bed while they are sleepy but awake. This won't work for every baby. If it doesn't work, you can try again when they are a bit older. If you don't like leaving them alone yet, you can stay with them until they go to sleep, but you will have to do this every time they wake up during the night. Place the baby in their bed during the day while they are awake and happy. This helps them develop a positive association with it.

You are going to go through some trials and errors while you are figuring out what is best for your baby. You might put them down in their bed, read them a book, and rub their backs for a bit before you leave the room.

Some experts will tell you not to nurse or rock your baby until they are asleep, even when they are very young. Everybody doesn't agree with this, so you just have to do what is best for you. The best thing you can do to create a good bedtime routine is to do the same thing every single night.

When Do Babies Begin Sleeping All Night?

This is dependent on your child. It usually happens right around six months, but all babies cannot sleep for eight to 12 hours without being fed during the night. This isn't saying that your baby will. Some babies will sleep for eight hours as early as a couple of weeks old, but most aren't going to sleep that amount of time until they get older.

Even if they don't sleep through the night, their sleep patterns will get more predictable after a couple of months.

Sleep Tips

We know that babies will have unpredictable sleep habits, which could mean a lot of sleep deprivation for many new parents. Keep reading to find some good tips on how to create good sleep habits for your baby. Your baby is going to sleep a lot. They will sleep between two and four hours every two hours night and day. Once they reach two weeks, you will notice that your baby is sleeping less during the day and more during the night. Many babies will sleep through the night by the time they are between four and six months old.

Naptime

Put your baby down for a nap every two hours. They might have problems falling asleep if you wait any longer.

Night and Day

By the time they are two weeks old, you can start teaching your baby how to know the difference between night and day. Remember, during the day, you have to interact with your baby as much as possible. Keep their room bright. If you have to do housework like running the washing machine, dishwasher, or vacuum, do it. Keep the lights dim during the evening hours. Keep the noises low. Make sure the energy in the house is calm. Never play with the baby during the night. Read, sing to them, etc. Don't get them excited.

Know The Sleepy Signs

When your baby gets tired, they are going to give you signs like being fussy, pulling their ears, or rubbing their eyes. My daughter would twirl the hair behind her ears until she fell asleep.

Swaddle Them

Keeping your baby swaddled keeps them calm. This makes them feel like they are still in the womb.

Play Calming Music

White noise mimics the sounds of being in the womb. It can help keep your baby calm. You can find white noise apps on most cell phones now, or you could buy a machine. Sleep can be hard for babies during their first three months. By six to eight weeks, they will start falling asleep by themselves.

Sleep Problems

Will I encounter any sleep problems during this age? You could, and it might be hard to see these problems while your baby is very young. You and your baby are trying to get into your own patterns and rhythms about sleeping. In the baby's first few months, they will need to be fed during the night with lots of cuddle time. If you can, you need to try your best to nap while your baby is napping during the day.

Your significant other could help you out by bringing the baby to you if you are breastfeeding. They can do some of the nighttime feeds if you bottle-feed your baby.

Learning to fall asleep and then stay asleep are skills that your baby is going to use their entire life. The following strategies can help you create some good sleeping habits for your baby from the beginning. Something to think about: there aren't going to be two families or babies who are alike. Look at the questions below to see if you can use the information with your child:

- Have you seen any patterns or trends in your child that might be a problem? If you have, what are they?
- What have you done to try and fix this problem? What worked? What didn't?

Things You Can Do
Below you will find ways you can help your child learn how to fall asleep and get back to sleep from their earliest months. Some of these might have been mentioned above, but they need to be said:

- Routines

A relaxing and loving bedtime routine can help your baby learn when it is time to go to sleep. Creating a bedtime routine and doing the same things over each night can help your child remain calm when it comes to going to sleep at night. Every family is going to have

30

a different routine based on their culture and their baby's needs.

- What is Happening In Their Life

There are going to events and situations that might lead to or make any sleep problem worse—being separated from a parent or getting a new caregiver. Exciting milestones such as learning new things could disrupt your child's sleep patterns. If these things do happen, by consistent and patient, above all else, keep that bedtime routine. With some patience and time, your child will get into the groove of sleeping through the night.

- Your Baby's Temperament

Every baby is going to create "self-soothing" skills at different points in their life and in various ways. The more intense and reactive your baby is, the more challenging it might be for them to soothe themselves. These babies will need a lot of help to get them calmed down again.

- Ready for Protest

While your baby is learning to fall asleep on their own, they might protest or cry. This is normal because this is a new change for them. It is essential to have a game plan to respond when they cry for you. You might want to look in them every couple of minutes, or you might not go in after you put them down. If you think something is wrong, please check on your baby. Going in and out of their room might make them more excited and upset them more. Think about your options, talk them over with your significant other, and figure out together the way you will respond. This can help you feel more prepared and follow through with your plan.

- Stay Consistent

Patience and time are required when you are teaching your baby any new skill. Staying consistent will help your baby know what to expect. If you change the way you respond daily, it will confuse them and make it harder for them to adapt. Once you can stay consistent, it will help your baby learn their bedtime routine faster.

Chapter 3: Three to Six Months: Getting More Sleep

By the time your baby gets to three months old, they should be sleeping around 15 hours a day. They will typically get 3.5 hours of daytime sleep between three to six-months-old that should be spread over three naps, with two to two and a half hours of awake time between the naps. Overnight, babies need to get 12 hours of sleep.

That's is a huge change from the sleep patterns that they had during their first three months. This period is one of the trickiest sleep periods for a baby. Their sleep patterns are going to change dramatically. This is when their sleep will become more like adults, with more distinct periods of deep and light sleep, and have more developed sleep cycles. This is when your baby's sleep habits become extremely important. Let's go over what is going on for your baby at this time.

The sleep cycle for a baby is constantly changing. During the first few months of their life, their sleep is very unorganized and is controlled by a biological urge. Some babies can fall asleep on their own once they get tired, and others may need help to drift off. This is when their sleep cycles aren't as pronounces as they will become. They also don't need a series of sleep cues or actions to help them get to sleep.

The biggest change to their sleep cycle will happen at around four months old. This is why it has become known as four-month sleep regression. It is likely the biggest change in their sleep that they will experience. Here's how it looks:

- The sleep cycle will become more organized, and their sleep begins to work more like ours
- Sleep has become more conscious, and it is a skill that will take practice for them to get right
- They are going to wake up fully between their sleep cycles instead of drifting between them
- If they rely on your to help them get to sleep by feeding, rocking, or so on, they are going to have to have them every time they wake between cycles
- Babies won't go back to sleep at the end of the cycle if they don't know how to self-settle, which will make them overtired in the evening

This is also a stage that is filled with other changes as well. This usually is when your baby becomes too big for the bassinet and gets upgraded to a crib. This may also be when you move them into their own room where they can sleep without interruptions.

Four Month Sleep Regression

Babies will experience several different stages during their first year where they may experience "sleep regressions," There are times when they will have to re-learn sleep skills because the parts of the brain in charge of sleep are now maturing and changing. Other regressions can be due to their development in social or physical skills around nap transitions.

They will wake up fully between their sleep cycles at four months and will no longer automatically drift between the cycles as they did before. Sleep is a much more conscious thing for them, and they will have to learn how to perfect this skill with your help. This is why if they get used to your rocking them or feeding them each time they go to sleep, they are going to need you to do that for them every time. That means you will be repeating this action every 35 to 45 minutes during the day and every two hours overnight.

This is not going to go away until they have learned how to self-settle. This means that they will be able to fall asleep on their own when they want. This act of self-settling won't happen overnight, as it is something new. They are going to need help and consistency to work on this skill. Please keep in mind that all babies will hit their developmental stages at different times. If they are about 3.5 months old and begin waking up every two hours at night, they have likely hit the four-month regression.

Stages of Sleep

In the first ten minutes of sleep, the baby has started to fall asleep and has entered a light sleep stage. A simple breeze or sudden sound can easily wake them up. Even laying them down if you are holding them can wake them up.

Between ten and 20 minutes, they have entered a deep sleep stage and are unaware of what is going on around them.

Between 20 and 30 minutes, they are deeply asleep. You will notice that their breathing is deep and regulated. This part of their sleep is the most restorative.

Between 30 and 40 minutes, they are starting to come out of the deep sleep stage, and if they happen to be over-or under-tired, they can end up waking fully at this point.

Between 40 to 45 minutes, their sleep cycle has come to an end. They will either wake up completely or go into a sleep cycle, beginning back at the light sleep stage.

At night, their sleep cycle will be longer than it is during the day. They will experience the deepest sleep between their bedtime and midnight.

About 45 minutes after you put them to bed, they can still easily be awakened, especially if they are over-or under-tired, uncomfortable, or sick.

Two hours after they have been put to bed, they will rouse out of their first sleep cycle. They are going to enter into a very deep sleep phase that will last until midnight. This is when they are less likely to wake up unless they become very hungry or they are sick.

At midnight, the deep sleep phase comes to an end, and they will enter a light sleep period. They are more easily awakened if they are uncomfortable, sick, cold, hungry, and over-or under-tired.

The baby's sleep cycle lasts two hours, so they will enter a light sleep phase at the end of these two hours and may end up waking up fully. This is the time when some babies could need help to go back to sleep.

By five AM, this is the highest chance that they will wake. If they do wake up fully, it can be challenging to get them to fall back to sleep, especially if their sleep overnight has been very restful.

Sleep Schedules

Routine tends to be seen as a very rigid word as it implies there is a rigid regimental pattern to the day. When it comes to young babies, we understand that keeping a rigid pattern to the day is not always possible, and it's not really something that you should try to do. It's only going to cause stress when you can't stick to it.

That said, an element of structure is important for toddlers or babies, but definitely around three to six months old. If you really think about it, we all have our routines we are going through each day. You may have a morning ritual you do each morning, like making coffee, eating breakfast, and reading the news before taking a shower. These are relaxing and comforting parts of the day because they are familiar. Babies are no different. This is why babies do so well when they have a reliable pattern to their day, which means that naps and feedings are predictable.

Sleep is just as important for your baby as milk is. It has a huge impact on development and growth. To encourage a good night's sleep, babies will need to take naps during the day.

Babies require a delicate balance of day sleep and night sleep. If they don't get enough day sleep, it will cause a buildup of cortisol in their body, which makes it harder for them to settle down at night. This can lead to them waking up a lot at night or waking up very early in the morning.

Basically, if a baby doesn't sleep well during the day, it can be very hard to settle at night. You already understand that tired or over-tired babies will be fussy, cry more, resist settling, and will have an extended unsettled period during the early evening that can go on for hours. So how much sleep should they be getting?

That's going to depend on their exact age. Babies vary in their sleep needs, and some are going to need more than others. You will need to assess your baby's needs and tweak them to suit your wee one.

Approximately, though, a three to four-month-old should be getting three hours and 15 minutes of daytime sleep spread across three naps. A four to six-month-old will need about three hours of daytime sleep spread across three naps. The best place for naps to fall is one in the morning, one after lunch, and then one in the late afternoon.

By five or six months, you may notice that they are starting to resist that third nap of the day. This does not mean you should drop that nap, though. Up until six months, this late afternoon nap is extremely important, even if it is short. This is because it ensures your baby doesn't become overtired at bedtime and then end up being unsettled during the night. Even a ten-minute power nap can help stave off any residual over-tiredness to help them sleep more restfully that night.

The length of their naps will vary during the day. The afternoon nap should be the longest at two hours because there is a natural dip in energy levels at this time. This long nap is important because babies enter REM sleep, and some amazing things happen during this time. These things include the creation of brain connections, a boost to their immune system consolidation of new memories and skills, reduction of cortisol levels, and the regulation of emotions and appetite.

Napping may be important, but having the right amount of awake time is also important. Too much can cause them to become over-tired, and too little with cause under-tiredness. Both can cause poor nighttime sleep and poor naps. This can lead to a grumpy baby and frustrated parents.

During these months, their awake time needs are greater than when they were younger. They are more aware of their world and love to experience visual stimulation, playing, and laughing. If you are still trying to put them down for a nap after just an hour of being up, you are going to be facing a lot of protests from them, or there is going to be a lot more feeding or rocking than there should be.

They need to have about two to two and a half hours of awake time between each of their naps. This is enough awake time to make them want a nap later on.

While it may sound like an oxymoron, your baby can oversleep. Sleep is a nutrient. It helps to sustain their social, emotional, mental, and physical development, but too much of a good thing is possible. The issue with this is, nobody thinks their baby is oversleeping.

Too much day sleep can cause them to wake up a lot at night and them being unsettled because they need more awake time. If you do find that your baby sleeps a lot during the day, then there could be something going on.

The number one cause of excessive daytime sleep is an illness. Illness can hurt their sleep routine. It can cause them to wake up too early from their naps or cause them to wake in the middle of the night because of discomfort. They could, however, sleep more than usual as a way to fight off the illness. If you have a six-month-old that still wants to sleep like a newborn, they could have an underlying issue, so it's time to visit their doctor.

Another reason for excess sleep is growth spurts. Growth spurts can make a baby or toddler suddenly start taking longer naps and sleeping later into the morning. This is especially true for newborns. During their first six months, you may find that they go through several sleepy spells where they like to sleep around the clock.

Reducing Daytime Sleep

With the fact that we have to find a good balance between awake time and nap time, we have to come to the fact that we will have to wake the baby.

While this can seem to mean to wake your precious sleeping baby, it is advised to do so if your baby is at risk of getting too much sleep during the day or if they end up sleeping too long in the morning to the point that they run into their lunch nap. This is true for the afternoon nap as well because you don't want it to spill over into their nighttime routine. It's better to wake your baby during the day than have them wake you up at night.

First, waking them in the morning. Most people recommend that nighttime sleep for babies should be from 7 PM to 7 AM. That means you need to wake them up at seven in the morning. If they have established their own regular waking time, make sure you wake them up at that time if they haven't gotten up themselves. This helps them get used to a regular sleep/wake pattern. When you wake them up at the same time each morning, it helps them to keep a predictable sleep schedule.

To wake them up, you would simply reverse what you would do to get them to sleep. Instead of getting rid of stimulation, you add stimulation by turning their white noise, opening up the curtains to allow some light in, and gently patting them and talking to them.

The Effects of Solids on Sleep

Between four and six months, your baby will start letting you know that they are ready to start eating solid food. A lot of babies will start eating solids at this time, and one of the main signs of readiness is that they wake more frequently at night out of genuine hunger.

There is a myth that says once they start eating solids, they will sleep better at night, but that's not necessarily true. When they start eating solids, the amount they eat at first is going to be fairly small and will increase over time, so the impact on their sleep isn't going to be noticeable right away.

You should also use caution around the choice of solids and the time you feed them. Lunch is the best time to start feeding them solids, and if they are under ten months, you need to be careful about giving them a lot of protein at dinnertime because this can cause them to wake up more at night. This is because their body can't effectively digest protein at night since their metabolism slows down.

Night Feeding

You may want to know when you can give up those nighttime feedings. The best answer is, it will depend on your baby. It is normal for a baby to need nighttime feedings until they have become well established on solid food. A newborn needing five or six feedings at night is probably what they need, but if a six-month-old wants the same number of feedings, then there may be an underlying reason. Hunger isn't the only thing that wakes your baby, so it is best to rule out other factors first before you start tackling night weaning.

1.   They got too much or too little day sleep
The first thing you need to rule out is if their night waking was caused by getting too much or too light day sleep, or if their naps don't hit at the right time during the day to help them sleep at night.

2.   Sleep environment
You need to take a look at their sleep environment. If you aren't using a white noise machine, maybe you should try using one to see if it helps them sleep.

3. Daytime calories

Ensure that they are getting enough food to eat during the day so that they don't require as much feedings during the night.

Once you have gone over these factors, you can look at the times they are waking up to be fed. If they are waking up every two hours and are about four months old, it is likely a settling problem, especially if they don't have an issue going longer than two hours between feedings during the day.

Catnapping

When you baby catnaps, it means they are only sleeping for a single sleep cycle, 35 to 45 minutes. This could be caused from them being under or over-tired or reliant on a sleep association. This is common for four to six-month-olds, and it can lead to an overtired baby at bedtime because they haven't had enough restorative sleep during the day.

Catnapping isn't bad or a problem and is a part of development that all babies will experience, peaking in this age range. That said, prolonged catnapping can affect your baby's night-time sleep because it can care over-tiredness during the day.

The best defense to catnapping is helping them learn how to self-settle. Babies will sometimes need to resettle during a nap as well to get a longer stretch of sleep. Resettling them during the nap is better than getting them up completely from the nap because it teaches them that they are going to need to sleep for longer periods.

Establishing Sleep Habits

This is a great time to start working on establishing good sleep habits. As a newborn, figuring out when to put them down for the night was simply watching them for signs of sleepiness. Now that they are older, you need to switch to a specific bedtime and set consistent naptimes to help regulate their sleeping patterns and habits.

A good bedtime to have is normally between 7 and 8:30 PM. Any later, they are going to become over-tired and will have a hard time falling asleep. They might not seem tired late at night and may even become lively and energetic, but that is normally a sign that it is past their bedtime.

If you've not started a bedtime routine yet, you should do so now. It can include any of the following:

- Giving them a bath
- Playing a calm and quiet game
- Put them in her pajamas
- Read a story
- Sing a lullaby
- Give them a massage
- Kiss them goodnight

Before you begin the bedtime routine, try to encourage a bit of quiet time by switching off the TV and doing some winding down activities. This will help them to relax and will set the scene for them. Whatever will work for your family is fine, just as long as you repeat it every night in the same order, and this includes the weekends. The routine needs to be kept to about half an hour long. Even if they aren't feeling well, it's a good idea to keep their routine consistent. Once they have gotten ten hours of sleep at night, you can wake them up in the morning to help reset their clock.

Let's wrap things up by talking about the baby sleeping through the night. Most will start to sleep through the night by six months, but let's look at what it means to "sleep through the night."

At some point between three and six months, the majority of babies will begin to sleep for longer stretches at night and then work their way up to about ten hours at a stretch. This means that if they go to bed at night and then wake up at four in the morning, then they are technically sleeping through the night. Most babies between four and six months will wake more than once or twice to be fed. By six months, and likely before, they will be ready to be weaned and sleep longer.

Self-Soothe

When you put them to bed while drowsy but not yet asleep, it will help them learn how to get to sleep on their own. This will help make them more likely to learn how to self-soothe and go back to sleep after waking up during the night.

If you hear that they wake up, wait a bit before you check on them. Give them the chance to learn how to settle back down on their own. If they need more help to get back to sleep and believe they are ready, you can try sleep training. There are different methods of sleep training like no-cry, fading, and cry-it-out techniques. What works for you will depend on your parenting style, beliefs, and your baby's needs.

Chapter 4: Six to 12 Months: Sleeping Through the Night

Between the ages of six and 12 months, babies will start having better predictable sleep patterns. They might begin sleeping between 12 and 16 hours each day, including naps for healthy development and growth. Some babies are still going to wake up in the middle of the night to eat. Each baby's sleep and wake patterns are going to be different. Some people might nap a few times throughout the day or longer during the night and not take as many naps in the day. As they get older, how many hours they sleep during the night is going to get longer. Try to find your baby's average amount that they sleep in one day.

A six-month-old baby can normally sleep between five and eight hours each night and take two to three naps throughout the day.

A 12-month-old baby will have the same bedtime. They might begin waking up at the same time each day, too. They will take about a two-hour nap a few times during the day.

When you put your baby down for a nap or at bedtime, make sure you place them on their back. If they do roll over on their own, you don't have to place them back on their backs. Their sleep patterns are going to change as they age. When they begin sleeping through the night, they might have time when they have problems going back to sleep because:

- There has been a change to the family's routine like new work schedule, holidays, or traveling
- They have learned a new skill such as pulling themselves up and standing or rolling over
- They are going through some separation anxiety
- They have a growth spurt
- They are sick or teething

It may take a couple of days or weeks for them to get back to their normal schedule. Although this might be frustrating, you need to be patient, consistent, and comforting to your baby. Ask other people to help you do chores, laundry, or cook so you can get some rest and focus on your baby to help them learn how to comfort themselves back to sleep.

There isn't an adult or baby who will sleep entirely through the night. We all wake up several times during the night. However, we have learned how to put ourselves back to sleep. You can teach your baby how to go back to sleep.

Creating a Healthy Sleep Routine

Place your baby in their crib on their back when they get sleepy but are still awake. This can help them connect sleeping with their bed. Tell them that it is time for sleep calmly. All babies are going to be different when sleeping. Some are going to go right off to sleep when you put them in their bed, while other cry or fuss. You don't have to rush into your baby's room every time they cry. If you wait a couple of minutes, you might hear their fussiness begin to slow and then stop altogether. Babies haven't quite learned how to settle themselves, and they are still trying; it is going to take some time.

As they play and explore more, they might become more interested in what is around them rather than sleeping. You have to be patient and consistent. It is going to take some time for your baby to learn when their bedtime is.

If your baby is gaining weight and growing well, they don't have to be fed during the night. They might want to since that is what they have always done, but they might wake up for food when they are hitting a growth spurt. This will normally last for a couple of days. Keep things quiet and calm, feed them well, and help them settle down again.

If your baby's cry begins getting more frantic and louder, this means that they aren't able to soothe themselves, and they still need some help from you. If this does happen, you can try some of these things:

- Pat or stroke their cheeks, tummy, or legs when you lay them down
- With your hand on them, quietly talk, sing, or hum to them

- Make your touch lighter and lighter
- Continue patting or stroking your baby. Don't ever pick them up if they start moving around or like they are waking up more.
- Older babies might settle down when you leave their room; give them some time to settle down. It isn't going to hurt them if they do cry for a little bit as they figure out how to calm themselves
- If your baby begins to cry louder, pick them up and get them settled how you normally would
- The next time they cry, try to let them calm down by themselves. This might take many tries before they figure out how to go back to sleep by themselves

If you are worried about your baby's sleep and you aren't getting enough sleep, you might be wondering about trying to train your baby how to sleep. Sleep training is a phrase that is used for various ways to help babies go to sleep and stay asleep. These come in various forms. Some are free, while others might cost you some money. One way is to just "let them cry it out." For this approach, you just leave your baby alone and let them cry until they fall asleep. Most parents find this way to be too upsetting, and they won't follow through. I could never let my daughter do this. I felt like I was a horrible mom when she laid and cried for a very long time.

Every baby can learn healthy sleep habits; it is just going to take some time and find the right approach for your family and baby. It doesn't matter what you decide to do; you just have to feel comfortable. Sleep is important to everyone.

There are some things you need to think about while you are helping your baby create healthy sleep habits:

- Do you have a regular bedtime routine that tells your brain that it is time to go to sleep? If you don't, you need to start one.
- Does your baby know how to calm themselves? Have you always calmed them down? If you have, you need to begin teaching them how to do it. It might take a few weeks before they get the hang of it. Some babies might take longer to learn this skill. Just give them lots of structure, warmth, and practice.
- What does the baby do at bedtime? If your baby has been breastfed until they fall asleep, they are going to need support and time to learn how to get to sleep by themselves. Begin with some small steps to help them go to sleep in their crib. Spend time during the day in their room while they are in their crib. You can be straightening up their room, picking up their toys, etc. You can sing softly and talk to them while you work. It is fine to help them settle in their crib if they get upset. You can pat them or pick them up and rock them. Don't ever feed them or breastfeed them each time they go to sleep. This means they will learn that feeding and sleeping don't go together. Don't let them

feed until they fall asleep. Cuddle them and then settle them into their bed.
- Is there anybody else who could help you with your bedtime routine? With some practice, other people can help them to give you a big break.

Bedtime

Having a calming routine after you feed your baby for the last time will help them settle down before bedtime. If you can follow the same routine every night, they will learn the signs of bedtime and will know what to expect. Routines at bedtime work best if they happen before your baby show you that they are tired. This can be done about seven or eight in the evenings. If you wait until they show you signs that they are tired, they will be too tired by the time you get them ready for bed. A baby who is too tired might have problems going to sleep and staying asleep.

Give your baby some variety by singing a different song or reading a different book, but the same pattern before going to bed will help them tremendously. Here are some ways to create a calming routine:

- Bathe them
- Put them in their pajamas
- Snuggle with them while you read them a story or sing a song

- Place them on their back in their bed when they are sleepy but awake. This can help them learn that their bed is where they sleep.
- Kiss them and tell them goodnight

If you are away from home, try to keep the same routine if at all possible. This could keep from upsetting their routine once you are back home. Each family is different, and you might need to try a couple of things to find out what will work best for you.

Naptimes

Babies are going to need to take naps. Naps give them the chance to rest while their brains grow. This keeps them healthy and ready to explore, learn, and play. Night or day, your baby is going to give you some clues as to when they are ready for bed. They might:

- Become still and quiet
- Lie down
- Have glazed eyes
- Rub their eyes
- Yawn a lot
- Get fussy
- Lose interest in their toys
- Lose interest in you

If your baby doesn't get an opportunity to sleep when they show you these signs, they could:

- Have problems falling asleep

- Become extremely fussy
- Become too tired
- Find an energy spurt and begin playing again

You need to plan your activities around their naptimes. Taking naps simultaneously every day will help your baby develop good sleep habits, which makes sure they get all the rest they need.

Self-Soothing

With some time, your baby can figure out how to self-soothe. This can help them go to sleep or go back to sleep when they wake up at night. It could help them soothe themselves during other times, too.

Your Baby Is Self-Soothing If They

- Fuss or grunt without being fully awake
- Stare at an object or spot for a couple of minutes before they close their eyes
- Rub their blanket between their fingers
- Make sucking noises
- Suck their thumb or fingers

You can help by:

- Make a gently humming sound that they can mimic. They might begin making the same sounds as they soothe themselves.
- Hold their hand gently
- Pat or rub their leg, tummy, or cheek while you are cuddling them

- If they are able to control their arm movements, they will begin doing these things by themselves if they get tired or upset. It might take them a few weeks to figure out how to do these things, but it is a skill they need to learn
- If they start fussing while sleeping, wait to see if they settle back down
- Wait until they are completely awake before you go to them

Just because your baby is learning how to self-soothe, it doesn't mean you take away your care and attention. Your baby is still going to need your help if they are scared, upset, or sick. Learning how to self-soothe will help them get back to sleep as they go through their sleep stages at night.

Six-Month Sleep Regression

Six months is a huge milestone for several reasons. It isn't just a baby's first half-birthday, but it might kick off a time of some major changes in their sleep, activity, and development.

Between four and six months, most infants begin showing some good progress toward sleeping longer and sleeping throughout the night. Sometimes this progress will hit snags, and sleeping problems might rear their ugly heads.

This is normally called sleep regressions. It shows a step backward or a stop in your baby's process toward normal sleep. Even though these don't last very long, they can be challenging for parents. Knowing some background about baby sleep strategies can help you during this six-month sleep regression.

How Does A Baby's Sleep Change?

When a baby turns six months old, they need to get between 12 and 15 hours of sleep each day. Many babies during this age begin staying asleep for longer periods of time. This is called sleep consolidation. Even though they normally nap a few times during the day, more sleep will shift toward nighttime, and many will begin sleeping through the night.

Six-month-olds will have a boost in their mental and physical growth. They will reach many developmental milestones during this time. Being aware of their environment will increase, and they will be more responsive to sounds, babble, and laugh more. They might gain some physical abilities such as sitting without being supported or rolling over. These factors might play a huge role in your baby's sleep habits and activity levels during the night and day.

The Cause of Sleep Regression

There isn't a clear reason behind sleep regression. As a baby grows, their development comes in unevenly, and this could cause times when their sleep hits a plateau, or it might get worse.

Many factors could affect your baby's sleep, and it might not be possible to find one single cause for their sleep regression. With their mental and physical abilities increasing along with being more aware of their environment, they might become more sensitive to disturbances, separation anxiety, or being overstimulated that could harm their sleep. Parents might be adjusting their sleep schedules or routines, and it might take your baby some time to get used to the change.

Will Every Baby Have a Sleep Regression?
Some babies will have a sleep regression, but some don't. In fact, some people might see an improvement in their baby's sleep, including longer periods of sleep, even though some patterns within a baby's sleep show that each baby is different. This means that one parent should never be surprised if their child experiences sleep regression or if their sleep stays the same.

Symptoms of Sleep Regression

Here are some possible signs of sleep regression:

- Waking up more at night
- Problems falling asleep
- Longer naps during the day
- More agitation or crying while awake

The amount of time these symptoms happen could change for every infant. Normal symptoms won't last for long as long as parents use some good sleep tips. Sleep problems normally work themselves out in a few days or weeks, even though improvements could continue for a longer amount of time.

How to Cope With Sleep Regression

If a sleep regression happens, it is a great opportunity for parents to see how they can approach their child's sleep. Even though there isn't a cure for sleep regression, the following tips might help you reinforce positive habits that will promote better sleep.

- Create a bedtime routine
- Have a regular sleep schedule
- Know the safe sleep guidelines
- Reinforces knowing night from day
- Minimize all distractions while our baby sleeps
- Help your baby fall asleep in their bed

Even if you follow every step right, your child might still wake up during the night. If this does happen, don't rush to them immediately. Wait a few minutes to see if they calm down on their own. If you have to check on them or they need to eat, keep the sound and light to a minimum and try your best not to stimulate them.

Separation anxiety might cause your child to cry when you walk out of their room. If this happens, don't take them out of bed; just try to comfort them by rubbing them and talking to them in a calm and soothing voice. When they have relaxed, you can leave their room and let them sleep.

12-Month Sleep Regression

By the time a baby turns one year old, parents are amazed at how much the baby has developed and grown. Other than getting bigger, being more responsive, being more active, most 12-month-olds have shown some great progress in sleep.

But children's sleep patterns can change during this age. Although babies might have begun sleeping through the night, they might all of a sudden have problems falling asleep or wake up a lot during the night.

If your baby seems like they have taken a step backward in their sleep routine, this is normally called sleep regression. Even though sleep regression could happen at various points in a child's life, it is common for one to pop up about 12 months.

Sleep regressions don't normally last long but knowing what can cause these and ways to handle them could help you support your child's sleep.

How Does Their Sleep Change At 12 Months

As a baby gets older, they normally sleep for longer periods of time. Most of their sleep will happen during the night, even though they will take naps throughout the day. When they turn one, they won't need as much sleep every day.

Most babies will begin sleeping through the night at about six months, but this won't happen with every baby. An infant's sleep development is very different, and most children's sleep patterns won't follow the same timeline. Parents can expect to see more and longer nighttime sleeping, but many won't be as fortunate.

These sleep fluctuations will happen along with other aspects of a child's development. A child who is one will shoe more emotional engagement, better communications, better cognitive skills, and better physical abilities like walking and standing. These, along with other milestones, might influence your baby's nighttime sleeping and daytime activities.

Causes of Sleep Regression

When a child turns one year old, some children will have a round of sleeping problems. This sleep regression might happen regardless of what their sleep experience has been.

Figuring out the main cause of sleep regression is hard since it could be affected by many things.

Because of the child's changes, it is normally hard to find one main reason why they might be having sleep problems.

Some causes of a sleep regression might include:

- Some children might have nightmares
- Adjusting to new sleep training, schedules, or patterns
- Teething and other discomforts and pain
- Separation anxiety that just builds up with heightened social and emotional development
- Overstimulation and restlessness are related to increased activity levels and physical growth.

Will Every Child Have Sleep Regression?

No, not every child will have sleep regression. An infant's sleep development changes a lot, and this makes their sleep patterns change, too. A study that was done found that about 72 percent of all one-year-olds would sleep about six hours at a time each night. Even though sleep regressions do affect some children, other parents might see their child's sleep get better or stay the same.

Symptoms of Sleep Regression

Sleep regression can take on many different forms, but the most common ones are:

- Taking longer naps throughout the day

- Not wanting to go to bed
- Crying being agitated a lot
- Being fussy
- Having a hard time going back to sleep after waking up
- Waking up more at night

Parent Self Care

Parents need to remember that they need to take care of themselves and get all the sleep they need. Although it is tempting to just focus on the baby's needs, healthy parents will be able to give the attentive and loving care their baby needs.

Part of this self-care will be not to blame yourself if your baby has problems sleeping. It is normal for babies to have problems sleeping through the night even after they have turned a year old. Knowing that your baby might go through some of these phases could help a parent set expectations and adapt to how their child is developing and growing.

Chapter 5: Welcome to Toddler Sleep

Your baby is now a year old, and sleeping must become easier now, right? While, in theory, sleep time can become easier, there is still a lot going on. Between the ages of one to five are the most important times for reinforcing good sleeping habits for your child. They are going to need a lot of sleep to stay physically and mentally healthy. Why is it that bedtime always ends up becoming a battle? A lot of toddlers will refuse to sleep all night because they find like for stimulaing, and at this stage, going against the norm is fun.

While there may not be an easy fix for children who never seem to be tired, you can help them calm down so that they can get the kind of rest they need. You have to take the time to come up with a regular routine and then stick to it. You have to make sure that you don't give them any type of wiggle room when it comes to bedtime. Get rid of screen time and sugary snacks before and try reading to them and bathing them. Before long, they will find going to bed much easier.

Toddlers need to get between 11 and 14 hours of sleep during the day. Up until age two, they will get those hours through a combination of two one to two hours naps a day and ten hours of sleep at night. After the age of two, they only need one nap in the afternoon plus ten hours of sleep at night. While toddlers are most well know for wanting to resist sleep, with your help, they can learn healthy sleeping habits by making sure their nape times and bedtimes are the same every day. This makes things easier because they will know what to expect.

Sleep Schedule

Most toddlers do better when they get into bed by 7:30 or 8. This is because kids who can fall asleep before nine will go to sleep faster and they sleep better through the night, waking up more rested. You can also expect a wake-up call at around six or seven in the morning. Some may wake up earlier, though there are some tools to help these early risers to help them hit their snooze button.

What To Do with a Resister?

If your child wants to fight bedtime, there are some things to keep in mind. The most important thing you need to make sure you don't do is threaten them or get into a battle of wills. This is only going to cause them to associate bedtime with punishment. If they insist that they don't feel sleepy, tell them they can play or sing quietly with a couple of their stuffed animals until they are ready to go to sleep. When you do this, it makes them feel as though they have won something, which makes them feel satisfied and will help them sleep better.

You can also switch the lunch to an earlier time and get their afternoon nap out earlier so that they have a longer time to play before bedtime. That way, once their head hits the pillow, they will be out like a light.

Why They Fight Sleep

Now that they had started learning how to talk, developed an iron will, and had a longer attention span, bedtime gives them a great chance to test their new skills. There are a few reasons why they want to fight sleep and some ways to overcome those problems to put an end to the battles.

1.   They Don't Want to Give In
Toddlers are going to say no, that's who they are. If mom is saying, it's time for bed, that couldn't possibly be a good thing. The trick this is to make them think it is their idea but letting them have a bit of say-so over their routine. Allowing them to pick between two pairs of pajamas, what stuffed animal they sleep with, and what book to read will help them accept that it's lights out at seven. Make sure that you decide on all of this before you get to bedtime. Negotiations can drag on for a long time if you don't control them.

2.   They Are Afraid That They Will Miss
        Something
Your social butterfly wants to take part in everything, except for the bed. To help make the transition smoother between wake and bed, you need to try and create a calm atmosphere by having a soothing conversation with them and giving them a bath. Once

you get them to be, do your best to stop any attempts to rejoin the "party" they think is happening. It can take a few trips back t their room than you would like, but they are will figure out that they aren't actually missing out on something.

3. They Want To Be With You
Separation anxiety affects kids of this age a lot, so if they bed you to stay in their room when it's bedtime, they aren't playing a game. To try and reduce this problem, partake in a neutral conversation about what happened during the day and what they might expect tomorrow. Make sure that these chats are boring and short.

Naps

The best option with naps is that they take two naps each day that last about one to one and a half hours. Once they are between 16 and 20 months, you can transition to one nap, keeping it in the afternoon and about one and a half to two hours long. Expect them to be crankier and sleepier as they get used to these adjustments. You can move their lunch back so that their afternoon nap can happen earlier as they get used to the new schedule.

When it is nap time, it is better to have a place that you have designated for sleep. Instead of letting them nap on the couch or in a stroller, you should make sure they nap in the bed. This ensures that they associate in a consistent place with sleep.

Sleep Strategies

You can use some strategies that will help you deal with bedtime. First, active days will give you a restful night. Make sure that they have had plenty of time to get their energy our during the day. This is going to get them ready for bedtime.

Then you have the bedtime routine. There is no mystery to this. All you need to make sure you have are the three Bs: bath, books, and bed. You can play around with what you let them do before bed, but once you find something that works for them, don't play around with it too much. If you add too much to this, the less shut-eye they are going to get. The most important this is to stay consistent.

Next, keep an eye on those pre-bed snacks. If they need a snack before bed, go with plain crackers and cheese and maybe a glass of milk.

You also need to cut out screen time before bed. All screens need to be switched off at least 30 minutes before it is time for their bed. You also have to make sure they don't have screens in their room. You should also avoid any type of scary material.

Co-Sleep and Tummy Sleep

While bed-sharing should not be done during their first year since it increases the chances of SIDS, bed-sharing with a toddler is up to you. That being said, that doesn't mean that co-sleeping is a good idea.

When you co-sleep, it makes it a lot harder for them to learn how to sleep well, including the best way to sleep alone.

Plus, parents who share a bed with their kids say that they have a lower sleep quality and quantity. It also prevents them from having any intimate time with each other. This is why experts agree that children are better off when they sleep in their own room and bed. They can sleep better, sounder, and you will also be able to sleep better.

As far as tummy sleep goes, the risk for SIDS is the highest during their first four months, so once they reach the toddler years, they can sleep in whatever position they want, and this includes the tummy.

Causes for Sleep Problems

There are plenty of reasons why your toddler doesn't want to sleep well. Let's dive into some of the reasons why.

1. No Routine

This is probably the most common reason why a toddler doesn't want to go to sleep and is the one that is most easily fixed. Coming up with a consistent bedtime routine will help ensure that they get plenty of sleep. Once they have gotten used to this consistent routine, it will make them fall into a sound sleep, and they will be less likely to resist this process since they will see it as a normal part of their day.

2. Bad Dreams and Fears
Whether they are afraid of the dark or afraid of the monsters under the bed, nighttime fears can be very real to them. You can pat them and reassure them that they are fine, but you shouldn't linger too much. It will also help them get back into their sleep routine if you don't hang around too long.

3. Illness or Vacation
You know how hard it is to get to sleep if you are sick or when you're in a strange bed. Now put yourself in your toddler's shoes, who is still just trying to find their way when it comes to sleeping. It is best to take a whatever-works attitude during these rough times to help them get to sleep. If that includes extra hugs, kisses, middle-of-the-night cuddles, and special bedtime requests are acceptable in certain circumstances. The important thing is to make sure you get them back to the regular routine as soon as you can.

Toddler Myths

People are full of "great" parenting advice. While they may be well-meaning, a lot of their advice is plain wrong. We are going to dispel some common myths that you could hear about toddler sleep.

1. A Night-Light Can Hurt Their Vision
This is wrong. There are generations of parents who have used dim night-lights in their child's room. Do they need a night light? Having a night-light in their

room can help you check in on them at night without having to turn on a bright light that could wake them up. Plus, many will feel safer if they can see some familiar things if they were to wake up around two in the morning.

This myth's origin comes from a study done in 1999 at the Children's Hospital of Philadelphia. They said that 34% of children who had used a night-light ended up becoming near-sighted. Over the next year, two new studies came out to debunk this claim. Ohio scientists discovered that only 16.8% of the children in the study who had been exposed to night-lights during the first two years had a chance of becoming nearsighted, compared to the 20% of those who slept in darkness. Boston scientists confirmed that there wasn't a correlation between vision problems and night-lights.

2. It's Normal for a Child to Sleep Alone
The truth is, who really wants to be alone at night. There are cultures where young children sleep with their parents or siblings for years. Parents are surprised to find that bed-sharing often increases as they get older. By three years, 22% of children will bed-share, and 38% of four-year-olds will bed-share at least once a week. Among preschools, 10 to 15 percent will bed-share. The important thing is to try to get them to use to sleeping on their own as much as possible, but don't be surprised if they want to share the bed with you from time to time.

3. Toddlers Sleep Through the Night
There are video studies that have found that toddlers
wake up during the night several times. We normally
don't know because they can put themselves back to
sleep without waking us up.

4. Toddlers Need Less Sleep than Infants
While their daytime sleep will decrease as they go
down to just one nap a day, a lot of toddlers will need
11 to 12 hours of sleep each night until they are five.
Between six and 12 years of age, it will only drop to
nine to 12 hours.

5. Toddlers Need to Get Rid of Pacifiers
It is comforting and normal for toddlers to suck. In
several cultures worldwide, children can suckle at the
breast until they are three or four. Pacifiers help
promote their confidence and increases their ability to
self-soothe during the night. Furthermore, a lot of
toddlers have a strong urge to suck. They should use a
pacifier rather than start sucking on their thumb,
increasing their risk of long-term orthodontic issues.

6. Sleep Has Nothing to Do with Their Ability to
     Learn or Their Health
Besides triggering a host of daytime behavior
problems like defiance, impulsivity, aggression,
crankiness, and tantrums, sleep deprivation can also
hurt their memory, acquisition, knowledge, and
attention.

Some studies have found strong links between kids
who sleep too little and health issues later in their

lives. What's surprising is a reduction of only an hour of sleep a night during this time can affect their learning abilities in school. Canadian researchers found that getting fewer than ten hours of sleep made toddlers and preschoolers twice as likely to be overweight, do poorly on tests, and be hyperactive.

7.   Kids Will Fall Asleep When They Get Tired
While everybody does tend to fall asleep once they get exhausted, some toddlers can become more awake. They can get giddy and start running in circles. This can often make it look as though they have ADHD. This can escalate easily. The more tired they become, the harder it becomes for them to fall asleep.

8.   A TV Can Make Them Sleep Better
A TV can become a huge problem. Almost a third of preschools have TVs in their room, with 20% of infants having one. A fifth of parents will use television as a part of their bedtime routine, but these electronic pacifiers are a bad idea.

A TV in their room can disrupt their sleep and make it a lot harder to sleep. Studies have found that watching TV before bed can cause sleep problems, including issues staying and falling asleep. Children with TVs in their bedroom will:

- Watch more television
- Go to bed 20 to 30 minutes later
- Resist sleep – they are more likely to fall asleep after ten

- Sleepless – they are more likely having a hard time waking up the next morning
- Exercise less
- Have greater psychological stress
- At a higher risk of becoming obese or overweight
- They can get hurt if they accidentally pull the TV on them

This doesn't mean you have to get rid of your TVs. Just make sure you are with them when watching television, and don't put one in their room.

Chapter 6: Teaching Them to Wind Down

As adults, we know we often have to wind down at the end of the day to get a decent night's sleep. Children need to do that too, but they don't know how to do that. That's where we come in. We have to teach them how to wind down. We've already touched on the three B's. That is a basic routine you can do each night with your child that helps them relax and go to bed. Children to have consistency in their life. These bedtime routines are helpful because they let your child know that it's time for bed, but what else can they do?

What about what you do with them before bath time? Evenings are one of the best times to spend more quality time with your family, especially once they are in school. When it comes to picking activities to do during this time, it is best to go with things that will help them wind down. The worst thing to do is have them do things that are going to get them revved up before trying to put them to bed.

It seems, though, that they act worse in that time before bed. We've all experienced children who are "bouncing off the walls." They fidget, act silly, screech with laughter, and rough-house. All of this can drive a parent crazy. This is all a part of being a child, though, but we still have to get them to calm down to go to bed or even to eat and do their homework.

Are They Acting Out?

Before we get into ways to help them wind down before bed, let's discuss what it means for a child to act out. When they start getting wound up, it can be hard to tell if they are just a child or if they are acting out. How can you tell if they are displaying normal behavior for their age group, or if the hyperactivity could be a sign of a bigger issue, like ADHD? One thing you can do is compare them to their peers. Comparison is not generally a tool you should often do, but it can give your baseline for how their age group acts. For example, when you look at a scout troop, you could see that one or two of them are a bit more difficult to handle than the rest.

However, that doesn't mean that they have a problem. Basics things in life, like sleep and food, can make a big difference. Have they been eating a lot of fried or sugary foods? Maybe they have gotten into some caffeine? Help them include more vegetables, fruits, complex carbohydrates, and lean proteins into their diet, and it might help them hyper behavior.

You may also think that not getting enough sleep will help make them drowsy and ready for bed, but that's not true. A lack of sleep can make a person hyper. That's why you must help them get a good night's sleep, ensuring they get around eight to 11 hours of sleep each night.

Bedtime Is Hard

If you take the time to think about why bedtime is so hard for children, it makes sense. They are just like us. They have spent the time learning, listening, and playing, and by the end of the night, they don't want to have more orders shouted towards them. These orders will often prove to be too hard to handle.

They likely feel like we do when we have settled onto the couch with a good book, and then we have pulled away. We don't want to get up from that comfy position because we've finally gotten the chance to relax. But here's the deal, we may understand and empathize with how they feel, but we also realize how important getting plenty of sleep is for improving a child's mood and behavior. So, how do we inspire them to get started with their bedtime routine and listen when the last thing they want to do is listen to more orders?

How can we bring the night to an end with a strong family bond full of love and positivity?

One of the healthiest and most effective motivators for children is to have a close relationship with them. Humans crave connection, and it is hardwired as a primary need. Most adults won't realize this, but bedtime creates anxiety for children. It signals a transition into the longest period of their day that they spend away from their parent.

If they have been through a bustling part of the day without a lot of connection, a child's stress can be increased as they haven't had the chance to meet their primary need for connection. A great stress reliever for kids is playing, and play serves as one of their main forms of communication. The play also parks laughter, fun, and creativity, which research has found has many valuable benefits to help a child calm down.

You have to get rid of the marching orders and demands right before bedtime and bring in some strategies that will have your children responding to connection, fun, and creativity.

Setting Them Up for Success

Active and healthy children need to have a chance to release some steam. Take them, with the entire family, to the park or to an indoor activity place when it's cold, and let them play. The entire family should get involved because when parents participate, you may find that it helps you sleep better at night. This might not be something you can do every day, but you should try to make some time for it. You can also plan some things to help set your child up for success when it comes to winding down.

- Serve Good Meals – Ensure your child is getting three good meals each day. They need to start the day with foods high in whole grains and protein and low in sugar. Blood sugar and hunger highs and lows can cause a kid to become hyperactive. Eggs and toast are a much better option than a toaster pastry.

- Teach Them Relaxation Techniques – Adults can benefit from these activities as well. Meditation, deep breathing, tai chi, or other mind-body exercises can help a child slow their thoughts and body.
- Take a Walk – When you have a young child, take them by the hand and go for a daily walk. If they are having a hard time settling down to do their homework, have them go for a walk or a spin on their bike.
- Make a Boredom Box – Hyperactivity is often caused by boredom. Create a box that has models, building blocks, art supplies, books, dress-up clothes, or whatever activities will often hold their interest.
- Use Music – Soothing music, like classical, can help a child to calm down. Try different types of music to see what will work best for them. Playing soft music in the background during dinner, homework, and before bed can help them relax.
- Give Them Fidget Alternatives – If they tend to become restless when they have to sit still for a while, have some activities that they can quietly do that won't disturb others, like coloring books, puzzle books, a stress ball, or other objects that can be manipulated.
- Calm Yourself – If you become angry, frustrated, or upset in front of your child, they can respond by raising their emotional level.

Do some deep breathing, or step away for a moment to regain your composure. When you can stay calm and react in a neutral tone, you will notice your child stays calmer as well.

With that in mind, let's jump into some specific activities you can use to help teach your child to wind down in the evening.

Avoid Overstimulation

One of the main reasons children will have a hard time winding down is that they are overstimulated. When you chase them around and wrestle them, it will cause their energy levels to increase, which will make bedtime more difficult. Overstimulation is the biggest enemy of bedtime. This is also part of the reason why screen time needs to be limited, especially before bedtime. The light of the screen and the content they are watching can affect their sleep quality. Exciting video games or dramatic TV shows can engage their brain and cause their body to release adrenaline. This can make it harder for them to fall asleep.

A less obvious problem with screen time is the impact that light has on our sleep-wake patterns. Most of these devices will emit a bright light. Exposure to this light during the evening can increase alertness. This bright light disrupts their circadian rhythms by suppressing the release of melatonin.

Color, Paint, and Journal

Your head is often whirring with a bunch of stuff you need to get out before you can fully rest. This is also true for children; drawing and writing can help them release these thoughts and make their worries less scary. For older children, you can teach them how to journal their feelings before they go to bed. When they are younger, you can encourage them to draw how they feel. It doesn't matter if anybody else can understand what they are writing about. The point is for them to release how they feel so that they can relax.

Ask your child to draw or paint of picture of something that they got to do today. Once they have finished their creation, make sure that you ask them questions about the other things they did.

Puzzles

Puzzles help children with memory development, fine motor skills, and communication. You can also come up with your own puzzle by taking an image and cutting them into different shapes that they can put back together. Doing puzzles can also help enhance their mood, reduce blood pressure, and lower their heart rate, which will allow them to relax.

Blow Bubbles

Blowing bubbles is even fun for adults, so take some time before bed to blow bubbles together. This is a great activity that keeps children engaged for a long time. It can help a child calm down before bed and work on other skills like focus and visual tracking. Some schools do this at the end of the day to help calm down children because it has a soothing effect. You can also work on their counting and ask them to count the number of bubbles you blow.

Story Time

If you haven't been using books as part of your evening routine, you should add them in. Whether they can read on their own or read aloud to them, reading each night is something you should get them used to early on. It's something that they can get used to doing throughout their lives. To make things more fun, try making them a reading nook or fort with blankets so that they have a quiet area to read their stories.

Another option is to allow them to read for as long as they want, as long as they are quiet and don't disturb anybody. This could mean that they read late into the night, but chances are, they probably won't be asleep even if they weren't reading. Let them read so that they can slip away from their worries until they can't keep their eyes open. If they aren't reading on their own yet, you can give them some picture books that they can enjoy until they slip off to sleep.

Pillow Talk

Kids love talking about their day. When you set aside a specific time to do that every day, it can help them reduce the anxiety they have when it comes to bedtime. This gives them the chance to get in their last few stories they would like to share with you.

Podcast, Music, and Audio Books

These are great ideas for children who can't quite read independently. When they have something that they can focus on and listen to, it helps them quiet their minds and bodies. They get to be transported into an imaginary world of stories that helps to distract them from their worries. It gives them something new to focus on instead of trying to get out of bed. Listening to calming and quiet music does the same thing as well. There are a number of free audiobooks and children's podcasts.

Play with Putty

This is a sensory experience that can help them to wind down because they will be sitting still for a bit as they play, and they get to experience the texture of the toy. You can also make the putty into various objects and shapes.

Stretching and Yoga

Children need to have something that will replace the stimulation, so some relaxation techniques are essential. Stretching and yoga are great ways to help a child relax. You can also turn on some calming music as you do this. Stretching not only helps to improve their flexibility, but it helps them to relax. Since most stretches are held for 20 to 30 seconds, this will slow their body down to help them relax. Yoga comes with the same benefits. You can also ask your child to change the names of the poses to add in some fun. Other relaxation techniques for a child are a warm bath, essential oils, and a lotion massage. You can let them choose a couple of different relaxation techniques to help them go to bed.

Pick A Happy Thought

Like adults, kids can lay in bed at night thinking about things. They can replay everything that has happened to them throughout the day or worry about the next day. As adults, we sometimes assume that children have it easy and that they couldn't have any worries, but they do. They need help dealing with those worries. Something you have them do before bed is to get them to think of a happy thought that they will focus on. This will keep the mind from simply spinning. These thoughts should be something simple like an ice cream sundae, swinging, jumping in puddles, or a sunny day.

Weighted Blanket

If they are having a particularly rough night and can't get calmed down, a weighted blanket is a great thing to try. It is like a soothing and warm hug. It creates a sense of comfort, and it has been found to be a great tool to use at bedtime. The important thing is to make sure you have the correct weighted blanket for their size.

Other Bedtime Activities

To ensure you have a lot of activities you can try using to help them wind down, let's quickly go over just a few more.

1. Talk about your ancestors or family tree
2. Have the family share stories
3. Take their favorite stuffed animal through their bedtime routine
4. Look through a photo album
5. Tell them an embarrassing story from your childhood
6. Make them a human burrito with blankets
7. Have them list the feelings they had that day
8. Exchange favorite memories from the day
9. Stick glow stars on the ceiling have them make a wish
10. Layout clothes for the next day
11. Style each other's hair
12. Give each other massages
13. Listen to an audiobook
14. Try to finger knit
15. Do a calming body scan
16. Have tea time
17. Color
18. Rock them to sleep and sing to them
19. Have a healthy bedtime snack

20. List ten things you are grateful for
21. Share the best thing and the worst thing from the day
22. Write a quick song
23. Build something with Legos
24. Play a board game
25. Do a puzzle together
26. Journal together
27. Use some lavender essential oils
28. Do some yoga
29. Try guided meditation
30. Do a shadow puppet show
31. Plan breakfast for the next day
32. Race to see who can finish their routine first, parent or child
33. Brush each other's teeth
34. Listen to a favorite song
35. Everybody picks an animal to imitate through their routine
36. See how many stuffed animals they can put on their bed
37. Swap roles and pretend to be each other
38. Have them lay on the floor, like deadweights, and try to put on their pajamas
39. Walk backward everywhere you go
40. Play a game, but make the rules the opposite of what they are
41. Try not to laugh during bedtime
42. Pick crazy pajamas
43. Communicate using only hand signals and gestures
44. Make up a knock-knock joke
45. Read a story in a silly voice

46. Have a no talking only singing rule
47. Play "Simon Says" during their routine
48. Create a bedtime story where somebody in the family is the main character, and they have to guess which one
49. Share your five favorite things about them
50. Get the family together and have a tooth brushing party where you have music and dance while brushing your teeth
51. Pick out one another's PJs, and parent and child put them on at the same time

Everybody in the family has done their best during the day, so make sure the end of the day has a great ending. When you ensure you're responsive to your child's developmental and emotional needs for connection and play at this time of day, it will help make bedtime easier for everybody. It also allows you to make sure that the day is ended on a positive note, with love and peace.

Chapter 7: Have a Great Nap

You know your child must have a good nap. When it comes to naptime, though, you are faced with tantrums, excuses, and flat-out refusals to take a nap. Just know that this stage is not going to last forever. All of your efforts to get them to sleep are going to pay off. Benefits for toddlers and babies who sleep the recommended amount of time during the day in naps include better memory, attention span, better physical health, and better mood.

So what can you do when you help your child take a nap each afternoon to reap the positive benefits? While there isn't a quick fix, there are some things you can do to help improve their naptime.

Create A Routine

Children have a clock that will tell them when they are tired and hungry. However, they don't know how to satisfy those needs on their own. They had to nap because if they skip a nap, they are more likely to not sleep well at night. This is why naptimes need a routine, just like bedtime does. If you find that your 11-month-old had a great day when they got up at eight, took a nap at 10 AM for an hour, and at 2 PM for two hours, then make a routine of that.

Pay Attention To Signs

You must tune into the little clues your child gives you when they are getting sleepy. If you can catch them early on, you have a better chance of getting them to sleep. These signs can include fussiness, rooting even after they have finished nursing, finger-sucking, yawning, and eye-rubbing. It's best if you try to keep them awake while they are feeding and put them down for a nap once they are actually sleepy but not asleep.

Use The Bedroom

There are a lot of parents who like to let their child nap wherever, like the carrier, car seat, or stroller. Unless you don't have any other choice, though, you need to make sure that they take their naps in their crib. The best environment for sleep is a quiet, cool, and dark place. Even if you can't put them in their regular crib, you can create a sleep sanctuary in other rooms and put them in a portable crib. The goal is to create a soothing environment that will help them sleep.

Once you have found a cool spot, do your best to block out as much light as possible. If you are using their nursery, then it should already be set up for that. You can also turn on their white-noise machine. Try to head off any possible loud noises. If you know the dog barks when the mail comes, put the dog somewhere where they don't see the mail carrier. Do friends and neighbors drop by often? Put a note on your door telling them when to come back. If you are okay with them coming in while the baby is napping, ask them to call you to let you know they are there so that they don't knock and wake the baby.

Keep Them Engaged

The best way to make sure they nap well is to keep them engaged when they are awake. Make eye contact with them, or sing to them when you can. If you are talking on the phone, then pretend to be having a conversation with them. Taking a trip to the store right after they have breakfast can be an adventure when it comes to the sounds and sights they will experience. Toddlers and preschoolers need to get as much fresh air as possible and to get their energy out at the park. When it's rainy or too cold, you will have to permit them to do this inside. This could be dancing around to music, taking out the spoons and having them count them as they put them back in, or a jumping-jack challenge.

Let Them Fall Asleep

Just like with nighttime, you need to encourage your child to go to sleep on their own. It's important not to get stuck in the habit of taking extreme measures to help them fall asleep. These extreme measures could include putting them in a car seat or stroller and going for a ride or walk when they nap, or letting the nurse during their nap. Also, you should avoid holding the pacifier in their mouth when they can't sleep without it and are unable to put it back in.

If they start fussing after only being asleep for a few minutes of half an hour, don't run to them. That's what causes catnaps. Give them the chance to settle back to sleep on their own so that they can get their nap finished. Most of the time, they will settle back down.

Massage Them

A great method to try to get your restless baby to get to sleep during their nap is to use touch. Do whatever you can to make them as comfortable as possible. Make sure that they are clean and they have a full belly. Then lay them in their crib and give them a light massage across the back and head. If they still at the age where you have to put them to sleep on their back, rub their belly instead.

This massage helps to increase the bond between a child and their parent. It also helps to increase their melatonin levels, which will improve their sleep cycle. This massage doesn't need to last forever, either. A minute of light touch should be enough to get them to sleep.

Set The Stage

Much like keeping nap time similar to bedtime, start turning down the lights and making things quiet the closer it gets to nap time. Create a wind-down period for them about an hour before they need to go down for their nap. You don't have to get rid of screens as you do at night but turn the volume way down. Keep any verbal discussion quiet and calm, as well. This method works really well for pre-K kids and toddlers. For babies, this could be speaking quietly to them, singing a bit before picking them up, and then take them to their room for the pre-nap routine.

Try Story Time and Meditation Apps

You can use apps like Stop, Breathe & Think Kids and Nighty Night as an interactive way to help kids relax for a nap. With Nighty Night, children hear a narration over the sound of a farm full of animals as they each fall asleep, which encourages them to do the same. The other app helps teach kids how to meditate away from their busy day and to get them into a state of relaxation. You can also use storytelling apps to help get them to take a nap.

Creating a Good Routine

Before we dive into the logistics of creating a good nap time routine, remember that these routines need to change with their needs. When you have a newborn, they will be taking three to five naps a day or more. Most of these naps will run into each other with feedings between. There isn't a clear wake and sleeping period.

By four to six months, their wake and sleep period become more defined. They will take two to three naps a day. By six, up to a year old, they will have two naps during the day. While every baby is different, they will often fall into similar sleep patterns. Before three months old, creating an exact nap schedule can be a futile attempt as it could end up interfering with breastfeeding by impacting your milk supply.

Once they have moved beyond the newborn stage, you can start to make those naps a natural part of the day. You can use the following steps to create a nap time routine.

1.   Get Them Dressed
When they are still little, you can swaddle them for nap time up until they are ready to roll over. Once you can't swaddle them anymore, put them in a sleep sack or some comfy clothes. You should also use a nighttime diaper so that wetness doesn't wake them too early.

2.   Give Them a Pacifier
To help reduce SIDS risk, the AAP recommends that you give them a pacifier whenever they sleep. If they aren't too keen on pacis, continue to offer them one anyway when they start a nap. It could help soothe them, but it's not a big deal. They don't want it.

3.   Pretend It's Bedtime
Use the same sequences of actions that you go through before bedtime. This could be "dinner," putting on PJs, reading a book, and turning off the lights. After around a week of this, you should be able to ease up some of the pre-nap routines so that it's not so extensive.

Here's a sample nap time schedule that you may follow with your baby.

Four to Eight Months – two to three naps each day. If your baby wakes up at eight in the morning, your day could go like this:

- 8– wake up
- 8:30 - breakfast
- 9:30– the first nap
- 10:30– wake up from a nap
- Noon – lunch
- 12:30– second nap
- 2:30– wake up from a nap
- 4:30– third nap
- 5:30– wake up
- 6:30– dinner
- 7 to 8– bedtime

Nine to 14 Months – one to two naps each day. Again, if they wake up at eight, their day could go like this:

- 8– wake up
- 8:30 - breakfast
- 10– the first nap
- 11– wake up from a nap
- Noon – lunch
- 2– second nap
- 4– wake up from a nap
- 6:30– dinner

- 7 to 8– bedtime

15 to 18 Months – one to two naps each day. Their sleep schedule may look very similar to the last, but they may stay awake longer in the morning before their first nap.

- 8– wake up
- 8:30 - breakfast
- 11– the first nap
- Noon – wake up
- 12:30– lunch
- 3– second nap
- 5– wake up
- 6:30– dinner
- 7 to 8– bedtime

1 ½ to Three Years – one nap a day. Most of the time, these naps will take place just after lunch. Make sure that they don't spill too much into the evening so that it doesn't interfere with the bedtime.

- 8– wake up
- 8:30 - breakfast
- Noon – lunch
- 1– nap
- 4– wake up
- 6:30– dinner
- 7 to 8– bedtime

These are just suggestions, and you can create your own nap schedule for your child. Most children do tend to wake up earlier than eight, so keep that in mind as well.

When Naps Come To an End

There will come a time when you have to accept the fact that your child no longer needs or wants to take a nap in the middle of the day. At that point, you will need to switch over to make sure they are getting enough sleep at night. We may want them to continue napping, but there will come a time when it's just not going to happen.

These nap transitions have been happening since birth. During their first 12 months of life, they transitioned from napping pretty much all of the time to only two naps per day. After that, they will move down to just one nap a day. The age at which they give up naps altogether will vary. Some will stop taking naps by age two or three. Then others will continue to nap until age five. The average age for a child to give up naps is between three and four.

That window of when your child transitions from one nap to no naps is pretty big. While you may know the averages of when this happens, how can you be certain that your toddler is ready to give up naps? The following are some signs that you can look out for.

1.   Not Falling Asleep Quickly at Nap Time
If you find that your toddler is taking a lot longer to fall asleep at nap time than they used to and aren't all that tired when nap time rolls around, then naps may be a thing of the past. This is one of the big signs that your toddler could be ready to transition away from their post-lunch nap. As your toddler gets older, they will be able to handle more awake time. For example, let's say they wake up at seven. While a couple of weeks ago they were tired by one, as they get older, that might not be the case anymore.

2.   Taking a Long Time To Go To Sleep at Bedtime
Another sign is if your toddler is taking a long time to fall asleep at bedtime and doesn't seem all that tired when it gets to bedtime. This normally goes along with the previous one. Maybe your toddler has been resisting their afternoon nap, and instead of going to sleep at 1:30, they don't drift off until 2:30. This might mean that they don't wake up until four or later. This creates a problem because this later wake-up is going to affect their bedtime.

Of course, even if they do go to sleep at their regular nap time, they can still end up putting up a fight at bedtime. Why? It goes back to the fact that they can handle more awake time now. Eventually, that afternoon nap will be too much afternoon sleep and will affect his bedtime.

3.   Skipping Naps
If they end up skipping their afternoon nap entirely, but they don't seem any worse for the ware, then they

may be ready to give up their naps. If they are skipping naps and you don't notice them become cranky, and they don't get too exhausted by early evening, then this is a sign you should start transitioning them away from the afternoon nap.

Keep in mind that these signs can seem like problems that the parents need to solve. While this may be true for the toddler who has always had nap issues, these can be signs that you need to cut out their nap. Most of the time, all you will need to do is phase nap out, and then the sleep problems will resolve on their own.

If you aren't certain if your child is ready to make the transition away from naps, look at the opposite. If they miss their nap, do they get cranky by early evening? Sleepy children become hyperactive, irritable, and sometimes mean. This could mean that they aren't ready to give up that nap if they show their normal signs of sleepiness by early afternoon, especially after lunch. If they are rubbing their eyes, yawning, and getting fussy, then they probably do still need that nap.

This nap transition can be a bit tricky. The transition is going to look different for every child. Some can give up the nap on day one and will never regress back into a nap. Others will need a more gradual transition.

For example, you may find that they go three days without taking a nap, but on day four, they need one. This can go on for a while and can change from every other day to every three days, to even once a week. Let this happen naturally, and don't try to force things. It is best if you use your toddler's cues to guide you.

If they aren't showing any signs of being tired at nap time, then don't force them to sleep. Instead, have them practice rest time. This means you can put them in their bed or room with some toys and books and ask them to play quietly for an hour. This will provide you with a break and helps them learn how to entertain themselves. If they do end up getting sleepy and are in that quiet environment, they can lie down and sleep.

You may also need to adjust their bedtime during the start of this transition. The overall sleep amounts for a two-year-old need to be 12 to 14 hours, so they still need that even if they aren't napping. For a three-year-old, they need 11 to 13 hours. That means once the naps are gotten rid of, you may need to put them to bed a bit earlier, and they may get up a bit later in the morning.

With those rest time toys, for when naps are gone, try picking out toys that they only get to use during this time. Before rest time, let them pick one or two for that day. Once the rest time is over, they will have to put those back. They only get to use them during rest time, making rest time more fun and appealing.

Books are a good idea for rest time toys. Make sure you have plenty of books that will entertain your toddler and are appropriate for their age group. Puzzles and latch boards are also good. Not only do they stimulate the mind, but they come in a lot of fun colors that will keep their attention. Little People are also a great toy for children to play with during their rest time.

You can also ease them through this process by waking them up a few minutes earlier than you normally would. Once you have them sleeping only about an hour, you can try to drop a nap entirely once during the week. Eventually, they will have given up their naps entirely. Remember, turn the nap time into rest time. You are going to want that rest time.

Chapter 8: Sleep Schedule

Bedtime routines are a sequence of events that you do the exact same way each night. This can help with the transition from being awake to going to sleep. They can help your child feel safe, calm, and comfortable as they get ready for bed. Having a consistent routine can give your child a better night's sleep.

Developing a Bedtime Routine

Parents need to create a bedtime routine early in the child's life. You need to try to do this during the child's first year of life. About four months old is the best time because your baby is getting more sleep during the night with some naps throughout the day. They are starting to establish a night and day cycle. Children need consistency; in fact, they thrive on it. You have to create a schedule with specific times for naps and bedtime. It is important to put your baby to bed when they get drowsy and don't wait until they are completely asleep. Babies have to learn ways to soothe themselves so that they don't have to rely on you constantly.

Here are some tips to help you create an effective and healthy bedtime routine:

Calming Environment

Just like many adults, children need a quiet and calm place to sleep. Be sure your baby has a firm mattress in their crib, and their room temperature is set at a comfortable temperature. Their room doesn't need to be completely dark. If they do better with a night light on, give them one.

Bedtime Activities

If you decide to do any activities before you put your child to bed, it needs to be a calm activity. If it is a fun game or something that gets them moving, it might get them too excited, and it will be hard to get them calmed back down. Choose an activity that tells your child that it is getting close to sleep time. Most parents rely on the "three Bs:" bottle, bath, books. Some parents have found that their baby sleeps better after a slight massage or when they play some soft music. With some experiments, you will figure out what will and won't work for your child.

Happy Tummy

If your baby is full, they are going to sleep better and for a longer time. Anytime you are trying to get your baby to sleep, it is best to feed them before you put them down.

If your child is older, you can give them a light snack that includes carbs and protein. You could give them something like a half slice of bread and a piece of cheese. Carbs are going to make them sleepy while the protein helps regulate their blood sugar until it is breakfast time. Make sure to brush their teeth after they have eaten.

No Distractions

Babies and many toddlers will have a hard time settling down before bedtime, so you need to begin changing gears about 30 minutes before. This means you have to turn off the television and limit any type of physical activity so they will focus on relaxing things like listening to calm music or reading.

Stay Consistent

This is hard for some parents to understand, but if you are constantly changing your child's sleep habits and time, you are going to have a hard time getting them to go to sleep. This holds for both naps and nighttime. Other than special occasions like vacations, birthdays, or holidays make sure your child remains on your schedule, and you go about your daily routine. If you can create healthy sleep habits now, are your child will benefit from them in years to come.

Tips to Get Your Child on a Good Sleep Schedule

If your child is staying up past midnight and they don't wake up until the afternoon, they aren't alone. Children have been out of school, and they haven't been doing their normal activities, and most of them are off their normal sleep schedules.

If there isn't any structure to their day, it is easy for a child not to have a reason to get out of bed. If a child's sleep is off, it will have a huge effect on the way they feel during the day. Here are some tips to help your child improve their sleep schedule

Create a Morning Wake Up Routine

Having good sleep habits start with waking up at a decent hour. Getting them up by nine each morning is a good compromise when they aren't in school. When children begin waking up at a decent hour, everything else will follow, and they will be more tired when it comes to bedtime.

It is best to keep the same schedule each day of the week and not sleep in on the weekends. Varying their sleep patterns can be a problem for older children. You really need to be consistent each day is the key to getting the right amount of sleep.

Daily Schedule

I'm not saying you have to have a plan for every single minute of every single day. Having some kind of schedule can help keep your children on track. Give your child chores, make them read, or learn something new each day. They don't have to spend all day learning or reading; just 30 minutes each day will help. There are many free online resources.

Regular Meals

Having regular meals is related to sleep schedules. If a child gets up late, then they are going to eat later than normal. If they eat too late, they will be hungry too close to their bedtime. Make sure your child has breakfast and lunch at normal times to keep their hunger cycles early in the day.

Limit and Monitor Their Screen Time

Technology is the main cause of most sleep problems. You need to set clear rules about technology early in their lives and stick to them.

- All devices need to be turned off by 9 pm. This is what is keeping most children up late. If they don't have them, there won't be a lot for them to do, and they will be able to fall asleep easier.
- Devices can only be used in the common areas of the house, never in the bedroom
- Never allow your child to use a device until their chores or homework is done

Go Outside

Encourage your child to go outside, whether it is playing in the backyard, riding their bike, walking, or going to the park.

Many parents might be afraid to let their children outside during the coronavirus pandemic. Still, if they are staying in their backyard and aren't around other children or people, they are going to be safe. Getting exercise throughout the day can help them sleep better.

Stop Taking Naps

When your children are over the age of five, they probably don't need naps anymore. Naps could be harmful to their nighttime sleeping. Even a short nap could throw off their sleep schedule.

Comfortable Sleeping Environment

Your child might find it easier to fall asleep in their bedroom if they know it is a place where they can feel comfortable. Here are some tips that might help:

- Create a routine, like reading or taking a bath
- Put a night light in their room if it helps them feel comfortable
- Keep it a comfortable sleeping temperature
- Get all devices out of their room

Children Are Flexible

With this pandemic, most schools aren't open yet, and this can put them and their parents under a huge amount of stress. Children are very flexible and resilient, so never feel guilty when you have to change their schedule. Try to find a reasonable schedule, and your child will feel safe.

Good Sleepers Go Bad

Have your child's sleep habits followed a pattern of "taking one step forward and sliding two steps back?" Just when you feel like you are making some progress, your child begins cutting a tooth or getting sick and is back to step one. It is enough to drive you crazy.

It is going to happen. You are going to have setbacks as your child develops their sleep skills. Basically, you have to create a base of good habits along with an established routine at bedtime. Any temporary problem doesn't have to keep them from sleeping through the night. Normally, the main mistake isn't getting them back on their regular routine. Suppose something happens that gets them off schedule, such as a new baby or a vacation, and you need to temporarily change things up. In that case, your priority needs to be returning to their normal environment and sleep habits, so these new behaviors don't turn into new habits.

To make sure these scenarios that rob your sleep are only temporary, there are some ways you can keep problems from becoming permanent and get your child sleeping through the night again.

Traveling

A friend of mine has a two-year-old boy that has slept through the night since he was four months old. She also has a 13-month-old girl who doesn't sleep all that great. Her name is Elizabeth. The family took several vacations during Elizabeth's first year and didn't handle the changes well. When they were home, Darla let Elizabeth cry herself to sleep, but on vacation, Darla would breastfeed Elizabeth and allow her to sleep with her and her husband.

That is fine for vacations because sleep doesn't always go as planned when you are away from home. It is fine to let the rules slide while on the road.

If you want to help, your child goes to sleep in a new setting and sits in the room with them. Do what you would normally do at home, like bathing, rubbing them, reading to them, etc. Do the same things you would normally do at home so you don't have to undo any new habits they might pick up while on vacation. When you do get back home, get back to your old routine. You might have to enforce them a bit more for a few nights until things get back to normal. If you give them a clear message, you can get back to the way things used to be easy.

Temporary transitions

While traveling, Ken and Mary always had the same complaint: the pack n' play was great for naps but not forgetting the baby to sleep through the night. Rather than getting woke up several times during the night by their baby identifying all the objects they saw in the hotel room, such as "light, light," they now bring a fold-away crib and put it in a separate room. Booking a suite might be a bit more expensive, but it isn't as expensive as paying for two separate rooms.

Once you get back home, don't do a night of transition. Yes, this means you have to stand firm even if your child tries to deny you. If at all possible, try to get back home before their normal bedtime. If your flight isn't going to land until 11 pm, just brace yourself before you take off that you are going to have a rough landing when you do get back home. Remember to stand firms so you can face those tantrums and tears. When you are on vacation, you can tell your child: "While we are here, you can sleep in the same room with Daddy and Mommy, but once we are back home, you go back to your big bed in your room."

Moving From Crib to Toddler Bed

Most babies will start climbing out of their cribs by the time they are about 35 inches long. This might happen anywhere between 18 and 24 months old. It might happen sooner. You just have to notice your child's behaviors. This might scare some parents as it could cause their "good sleeper" to turn back into a horrible sleeper. Getting your child transitioned from a crib into a bigger bed can be a nightmare. The child sees an opportunity for you to lie down with them to read to them or lie with them until they fall asleep, but what they really mean sleep with me all night. You might go from a bedtime routine that takes about 15 to 30 minutes to one that lasts for hours.

The biggest mistake that most parents make is they take down the crib too soon. Even though the child might be showing signs they are ready for a new bed, in reality, they aren't. Moving to a big bed isn't going to be an "all-or-nothing" concept. Give it a try for a few days or a week. If it isn't going too well, there is no reason to go back to how things were before. If you are thinking about moving your child to a big bed just because your child keeps climbing out of it, use a crib tent.

Don't Rush

If your child stays in their crib and is happy there, never rush them to move to a bigger bed until sometime between their third and fourth birthday. You might have a small creature wandering around your house during the night. Think about it from a preschooler's perspective: The crib's bars show their parent's authority. They might be thinking: "I can't get out of here; Daddy and Mommy put me in here." It is natural that taking away those bars will create a huge temptation for them to get out of bed and explore.

If your child has problems staying in bed, put baby gates in their doorway to show you still have some "control." People can still get into their room, and they can see out. But this keeps them confined to their room. If you can get the "prison analogy" out of your head, remind yourself that the worst thing that could happen is your midnight mover falls asleep on the floor of their bedroom. If this happens, you can just ease them back into the bed once they are asleep. Remember to close the gate when you leave the room.

Milestones

My niece Patty began sleeping through the night when she was only eight weeks old. It worried her mom when she began crying out at night about two months later. What happened? Patty had learned how to roll over onto her tummy while sleeping but she couldn't figure out how to get turned back over. Her mom would run to her crib and turn her back over before she go too upset. After a few nights, this new milestone didn't wake her up anymore.

When a child hits a motor or growth milestone such as walking or crawling, your child might regress in their sleep habits for some time. These normally don't last long and it is best to just do your best to ride them out. I promise you that these changes won't last long.

Daytime ONLY

There are some things that you can do to help your child sleep at night. If you practice some developmental habits during the day like helping them lie down when they are sitting or helping them sit after standing is one tactic you can use. After you know that they have mastered this skill fairly well, let them do it by themselves. Then, if they do cry at night because they pulled themselves up, both of you will know that they can lie back down by themselves. But until you are absolutely sure they can do this by themselves or if you are a constant worrier, you can ease into their room, help them down, tell them they are fine, and go back to bed. The most important thing is to not make a fuss or be too intrusive. There will come a point when you are going to have to let your child figure out by themselves.

Cutting Teeth or Sickness

It is hard on both parent and child when the baby is sick. The baby doesn't understand what is happening to their body and they only feel comforted when their parent is holding them. During these times, it might be best to sleep with your child. I know when my daughter had a fever, it didn't just comfort her to be beside me; it comforted me knowing I was right there if anything went wrong. Yes, it did take me a week or so to get her back in her crib but I wasn't going to sleep with her screaming anyway.

The hardest thing is getting them transitioned back to their own bed. It might be best if you go to your child and sleep in their room rather than bringing them into your room. You could put a sleeping bag on the floor of their room until they are well. By doing this, things stay consistent with them, and you are just conveniently on the floor should something happen. When the illness is over, the transition will be easier because they haven't changed beds.

The experts will tell you not to do this but if you just can't resist bringing your child into your bed, be sure they are really sick and not just trying to get to sleep with you. Never allow co-sleeping to go on unless that is your long-term choice. This can be reversed easily as long as it doesn't go on too long. The problem happens when their sleeping arrangement doesn't return to normal when they are better. This could cause behavior patterns that will be too hard to undo.

Fears and Bad Dreams

Things that make noise at night can cause a bunch of problems with sleep. It can keep your child from going to sleep or they might wakeup in the middle of the night. Some experts suggest you use imaginary things to battle imaginary things. A friend of mine created "monster spray." They just put water into a squirt bottle and told the child to spray their room anytime they thing a monster is hiding somewhere. There is more about this in the next chapter.

New Sibling

Your bedtime routine might be serene and easy... well it was until you decided to have another child. Your older child sees you giving this new baby a lot of attention so they are going to find ways to get your attention. They might scream and cry at bedtime demanding they get fed and rocked to sleep. These battles might continue until the baby starts sleeping through the night. If this doesn't work, you could try to put both children into the same room. The older child might feel more relaxed as they don't feel left out and alone. This might get them back to falling asleep in a matter of minutes.

Setting Ground Rules

When you are going through a transitional stage, every family needs a plan that will work for them. In order to make this happen, you have to have some ground rules. If sharing a room is what the family chooses, be sure your older child knows not to play with the baby or wake the baby up after the lights are turned off.

Try your best to keep your bedtime routing during any troubling or transitional times. If Mama normally reads Green Eggs and Ham, keep doing this whil Daddy takes care of the newest family member. You could swap out bedtime duties a few months before the baby is born. Anything you can do to keep your child's life consistent, the more peaceful you life will be.

Sleep Debt

A sleep debt which might have been caused by a later bedtime during summer months or you are phasing out daytime naps, might cause you some bedtime battles with your child. Losing just 10 to 15 minutes of sleep each day can have a huge effect. It could take you a month or more before you notice it because it will sneak up on you. There are some things you can do to repay this debt and get your good sleeper back.

- Create Naptime

If your child fluctuates between one and two naps each day, try to get them to take a nap in the middle of the day. Once you have established a naptime, it will help your child go to bed easier.

- Put Them In Bed Earlier

If your toddler has stopped taking their morning nap, make their bedtime an hour earlier to solve this problem. Their bedtime may have to be very early to help them get back into the groove.

- Watch Your Child

Stop watching the clock and learn to watch your child. You need to notice their behavior between four and five pm. You can ask yourself: "Is my child pleasant, engaging, calm, sweet, and adaptable or are they short-tempered, whiny, frustrated easily, and fractious?" If they are the latter, then you know that they need to be put to bed earlier.

Chapter 9: Sleep Issues

Sleep problems are normal with children, especially when they are still very young. Bed-wetting, sleepwalking, night terrors, bedtime fears, and insomnia can disrupt you're your child's normal sleep patterns. A child might not feel tired when it is their normal bedtime. Other children might have problems getting to sleep without a parent in their room. Some children wake up frequently during the night. They just suddenly wake up and they will toss and turn for a while trying to get back to sleep. Some might even wake up their parents.

Yes, it is frustrating to have your sleep disrupted and then realize you have to rush through your morning routine because both you and your child overslept. You might even have to deal with a moody, fussy child because they didn't get enough sleep. Don't give up all hope just yer. Most childhood sleep problems are linked to their behaviors during the day and their nighttime habits that you can help your child change. With some discipline and patience, you could help your child overcome their sleep problems, help them get to sleep and sleep through the night. This will help you get back on track for better sleep.

How Much Sleep Do They Need?

Children and teens normally need more sleep than adults if they want to function well. Below you will

find the recommended number of hours that children
need to perform well:

- Infants – 12 to 16 hours and this includes naps
- Toddlers – 11 to 14 hours and this includes
  naps
- Children: 3 to 5 – 10 to 13 hours and this
  includes naps
- Children 6 to 12 – 9 to 12 hours
- Teens – 8 to 12 hours

How to Know If Your Child Isn't Getting the Right Amount of Sleep

Children have problems controlling their moods when
they haven't gotten enough sleep just like adults. Not
getting enough sleep can affect a child's state of mind
and behavior. There are some cases where insufficient
sleep will mimic the symptoms of ADHD.

Here are some symptoms that can tell you if your
child isn't getting enough sleep:

- Get drowsy or "crash" a lot earlier than their
  normal bedtime
- Have problems waking up
- They fall back to sleep after you have woken
  them up for the day
- Fall asleep while riding
- Have problems following a conversation
- They seem "spaced out"

- Have problems concentrating during school
- Seem over-emotional, irritable, or cranky

If your child wakes up a lot during the night or they have problems getting settled down of the evenings, it might mean they are struggling with insomnia. This is the main sleep problem with children.

Insomnia

Insomnia is not being able to fall asleep or remain asleep during the night. This can result in sleep that doesn't make you feel refreshed. Most of the time, this problem will resolve itself with time. If your child experiences problems sleeping more than three time in one week for a few months, and you see that it is causing them problems functioning during the day, it might be insomnia or some other sleep problem

Causes of Insomnia

For most children, their problems falling or remaining asleep come from their habits during the day or the way they spend their time before going to bed. Consuming too many sugary foods during the day, watching television before bed might be enough to bother your child's sleep. Younger children are going to have problems making the connections between their habits and their sleeping problems; you are going to have to be the detective to find their problems.

There might be other reasons why your child might be having sleep problems and these include:

- Medication Side Effects

Some drugs like the ones used to treat depression or ADHD could cause insomnia in children.

- Caffeine

Most energy drinks and sodas contain caffeine that can keep your child awake during the night. You need to limit their consumption of these after lunch. What would be better is to stop letting them have these types of drinks if at all possible.

- Stress

This might sound silly to you and you might be thinking that children don't have to worry about stress but they do experience stress. Most of the time this stress gets triggered either at home or school. They might be having problems keeping up with their class, experiencing some issues with their friends, or they might be the victim of bullying. Stress at home could come from parents if they are having marital problems, a new baby, or changes in their sleeping arrangements where they are now having to share a room with a grandparent, parent, or sibling.

- Other Medical Problems

Your child could have a sleep disorder like restless leg syndrome, sleep apnea or they might have problems breathing from allergies or a stopped up nose. They might have eczema and they feel itchy, they might be suffering from growing pains. Make sure you keep your child up-to-date on their check-ups so their doctor can help you find any problems that might be hindering their sleep.

Insomnia Caused By "Too Much Time In Bed"

There might be times when your child's insomnia might come from having more time for sleep than they actually need. If this is the case, your child might fight you to go to bed or they might wake up during the night or too early. In order for you to find their perfect bedtime, notice when they start getting drowsy each evening. This is the time you should try to get them in bed. You need to begin their bedtime routine about 45 minutes earlier. If they are awake longer, they might get a "second wind," and then it will be harder for you to get them to settle back down.

Coping With Insomnia

Even though creating healthy habits ensures they will get better sleep, and this is useful for any age, it is very important for older children and teenagers.

- Make Sure Bed Is For Sleeping Only

If at all possible, encourage your child to only use their bed for sleeping and their bedtime rituals like reading a book. Don't let them do their homework on their bed. If you do, this can cause them to associate their bed with activities other than relaxation and rest. Also, don't use their bedroom for time-outs or they will begin associating it with punishment.

• Their Bedroom Needs to Be Comfortable

Many children sleep better in a cooler room that is around 65 degrees. If there is a lot of ambient noise where you live, use a white noise machine, run a ceiling fan, or use a sound machine to mask some of this noise. Be sure your child's bed isn't covered with toys as this could distract them at bedtime.

• Keep The Same Schedule

Try your best to keep the same schedule even during the weekend. This makes it easier for your child to go to sleep and wake up naturally. Adolescents shouldn't have to sleep more than an hour past their normal wakeup time on weekends. If this does happen, this shows that they aren't getting the right amount of sleep during the week.

• Make Sure Your Child Isn't Hungry

Never let your child go to bed hungry. Give them a light snack of a banana and some warm milk before they go to bed. DON'T feed them a heavy meal within a hour or so of their bedtime as this could keep them awake.

• Keep Them Active

Getting regular exercise can prevent restlessness during the night. They need to be active for at least one hour during the day. Try to keep them from doing

any vigorous activities three hours before going to
bed.

- Expose Them To Natural Light Each Morning

Opening their curtains or blinds can help your child
wake up. This shows them that the day has started.

- Watch Their Naps

Children need no less then four hours between their
sleep periods before they are tired enough to go back
to sleep. Even though their naps might be different, be
sure your child doesn't sleep too long or have a nap
too close to their bedtime.

- Limit Electronics

The blue light that comes off video games, tablets,
phones, and televisions could disrupt their body's
sleep and wake cycle and this makes it harder for
them to get to and stay asleep. Turn off these devices
one hour before their bedtime and don't allow your
child to keep them in their room.

- Quality Time

You need to spend some quality time together. Some
children want to stay up late because they want more
attention from their parents. If both of their parents
work during the day, evenings are the only time they
have to spend with you. Just talking to them about
their friends or what they did during the day will go a
long way for most children. If your child is under one,

take some time to just read to them, sing to them or interact in a gently way to help them wind down at night. Be sure you make eye contact with them.

Handling Other Sleep Problems

Other than bedtime routines and daytime habits, children could experience other problems that keep them from sleeping through the night. Wetting the bed, sleepwalking, night terrors, bad dreams, or being scared of the dark are some problems that some children have problems with. Most children outgrow these things fairly quickly and there are lots of ways you can address their sleep problems to make sure that both of you get a good night's sleep.

Sleep Anxiety and Fears

At some point in their childhood many children will experience a fear of going to bed or the dark. Most younger children have problems separating what is in their imagination and what is real. Even though the idea of monster in the closet or under the bed seems silly to you, it can be extremely frightening to a child. Even though it is important to allow your child to express their fears without making fun of them, it is important to not support all of their worries. Rather than using "fairy dust" to scare off the monsters or waving around a magic wand to get rid of ghosts, you would be better off explaining to your child how their imagination could trick them into thinking that normal things like a creaking door or shadows are something scary.

• Try To Understand Their Fears
Acknowledge your child's fears and try to empathize with them before you tell them that their worries are separate from reality and nothing bad will happen to them.

• Night Lights
If you want to give your child some extra security at night, put a night light in their room. Just make sure it isn't too bright as to disturb their sleep.

• Security Object
Allow your child to sleep with a security object like a special blanket or toy. Letting a pet sleep with them could help keep their fears at bay as long as it won't disturb their sleep.

• Explore Their Bedroom
Take time during the day to explore their bedroom with them. Let them look under their bed and check their closet for any "monsters." Talk about their fears in the daytime rather than at night could help boost their self-confidence and keep them calmer at night.

• Help Them Stay In Bed
Even if your child wakes up during the night, encourage them to remain in their own bed. You need them to learn that their bed is safe. You might have to

sit with them while they are going to sleep instead of taking them out of their bedroom

Night Terrors

These episodes are characterized by intense fear, screaming, and flailing during sleep. Yes, it is very disturbing to witness and watch as your child is having night terrors, it normally isn't a cause for alarm. These are usually produced by stress, medications, not enough sleep, or changes to their sleep environment. Most children will outgrow these by the time they hit their teen years. These are not like nightmares that we will talk about in a minute. Your child will stay asleep during night terrors. They probably won't even remember the event the next day.

Night Terror Symptoms

- Walking around
- Sitting up in bed
- Sweating
- Fast heart rate
- Heavy breathing
- Screaming
- Kicking and thrashing around in the bed

Handling Night Terrors

If you try to wake your child from a night terror, it could do them more harm than good. Try your best to gently get them back into bed if they are walking around or you can just sit with them and calmly talk to them until they go back to sleep. You can hold their hand or pat them on the back. Most of these terrors won't last but just a few minutes.

Even though there isn't a cure for night terrors, you can take some preventative measures to make sure your child is safe. If they walk around during their night terrors, make sure any door that leads to the outside is locked with a safety chain so your child can't unlock it to get outside. If their bedroom is on the second floor of the house, place a child safety gate at the stairs so they don't fall. Move any breakable or dangerous objects from their vicinity.

You can help your child by asking them if they are having any problems. Just talking about problems can help reduce tensions. Having a relaxing bedtime routine can also help reduce their stress. Add some lavender essential oils to their bath can help relax them before bed. Don't let them have any caffeinated drinks after lunch time. If you notice the night terrors happen about the same time each night, try to gently wake your child up about 15 minutes before to see if this helps. Sit with them until they go back to sleep.

Nightmares

Once a child gets to their preschool years, they might develop a fear of the dark. This can also lead to nightmares. Any feelings or problems that they are dealing with during the day could turn into bad dreams at night. Along with talking about the bedtime anxiety and fears that we covered above, it is important to talk with your child about any changes that they are going through. Changing schools, moving into a new house, parents getting a divorce, or getting a new sibling can bring about a lot of uncertainty in their small lives and cause nightmares. It doesn't matter the circumstance or age, take some time every day to talk to them and know what is happening in their lives. Make sure you talk through any problems that they might be having with friends, school, or at home. If they wake up after a nightmare, help them realize that it wasn't real and don't dwell on the details about the dream too much. Focus on getting them back to sleep.

Sleepwalking

This doesn't just involve getting out of bed and walking around. Most sleepwalkers will talk, sit up, and make movements like rubbing their eyes or fumbling with their clothes. Even though their eyes might be open, they might have a glassy appearance. Because they are actually still asleep, they aren't going to see things the same way as they do when they are awake. Yes, this kind of behavior might alarm you, they aren't aware of the things they are doing and they probably won't remember it the next day.

Causes

Some factors that might cause sleepwalking include medications, stress, illnesses, irregular sleep schedules, and lack of sleep. There is normally no need to see their doctor unless this happens often, involves risky behaviors, or results in your child sleeping throughout the next day.

Having a regular sleep schedule and sticking to it is usually enough to get rid of this problem. You could help reduce their stress by doing some relaxing activities before they go to bed at night. Have them use the bathroom before they wind down, since a full bladder can cause sleepwalking.

Keeping Your Sleepwalker Safe

NEVER try to wake up a sleepwalker. This can scare them. Try to gently guide them back to their bed. Be sure all doors and windows are locked and put safety chains on doors so your child won't be able to open the door. If your house has more than one level, place child safety gates at the top of the stairs to keep them from falling. Get rid of any objects that are breakable or sharp and make sure all clutter and toys have been picked up off the floor.

If your child shares a bedroom with a sibling, never allow them to sleep in the top bunk. Even though sleepwalking will stop by the time they are a teenager, keep the car keys out of their reach.

Bed-Wetting

Even though your child might use the bathroom without any problems during the day, some younger children might have problems controlling their bladder during the night. This can be very stressful and humiliating to them. Bed-wetting normally happens in children between the ages of two and four. It could continue into their school years, too. If both parents were known to wet the bed, the child probably will be, too.

Some other causes of bed-wetting could include:

- Their body produces too much urine at night
- They are constipated since full bowels put too much pressure on the bladder
- You child sleeps too deep and their bladder doesn't wake them up in time
- It could be a response to exhaustion, illnesses, changes in the home, or stress
- Your child's bladder hasn't developed enough to hold their urine for the whole night. Communication between their bladder and brain might not have formed fully.

Helping Your Child Cope

Although your child knows they aren't at fault when they wet the bed usually make them feel guilty or embarrassed. They might feel reluctant about staying the night at someone else's house or going to camp.

Make sure they know that you don't blame them and put a rule in place that nobody in the family teases them about it. If another family member wet the bed, it might make them feel better to know you had the same problem. Here are some things that you could do to help them manage the situation:

- Set an Alarm

If they keep having problems, ask their doctor about an alarm. These will detect any wetness and will wake up the child so they can get to the toilet. This might be helpful for children who are deep sleepers.

- No Fluids Before Bed

Don't give them any fluids three hours before they go to bed unless it is a small amount of water. Remind them to use the bathroom before they get in bed.

- Reward System

Set up a reward system for when they sleep through the night. Make them a chart and give them a sticker to put on the chart for every night they stay dry. If they make it through a week without having an accident, give them a "prize."

- Have Them Change the Sheets

When they do have an accident, have them help you change their sheets. Tell them that it isn't a punishment it is just teaching them responsibility.

- Use A Mattress Protector

Buy a mattress protector that has a "rubber" backing to keep the liquid from getting to the mattress. If this isn't an option, you could use puppy training pads on top of the sheet.

When to See Their Doctor

If your child has been successfully potty trained for six months, and then they begin wetting the bed, it might point to a medical problem that needs a doctor's attention. This might happen if the bed-wetting happens along with some other changes in your child like:

- Still wetting the bed when they are seven
- Their ankles or feet swell
- Having accidents during the day
- Pink or cloudy stains in their underwear
- Burning or pain when they urinate

Constant bed-wetting, especially when the child is over seven or they had outgrown it might be a sign of sexual abuse.

Conclusion

I would like to thank you once more for reading through this book. I hope that you have found the information helpful, and can enjoy many restful nights in the future. Whether you are a parent looking for a way to help your child sleep, or if you are getting ready for your first child, I hope these tips will help you out.

It can be tough raising kids. Sleep is probably one of the hardest things that kids seem to have a problem doing. For the most part, all they need is a good bedtime routine that will help them wind down before going to bed. There are times, though, where it may require a bit more work. If you use the information provided, and you don't see improvements in their sleep, then it may be time to talk to their doctor. Above all, be patient with yourself and your child. You will get a full night's sleep again, and so will they. Stick with it, you'll see the results.

Lastly, if you found any part of this book helpful, please leave a review on Amazon!